What is the HCG + 500 Calorie Weight Loss Cure?

The **HCG + 500 Calorie** 'protocol,' as it's discoverer, **Dr. A.T.W. Simeons** called it, is an amazing, but as yet unheralded, discovery for the **treatment** and **veritable cure** of 'obesity.' **HCG** is the mercifully short acronym for the tongue twisting, scientific name for the hormone **Human Chorionic Gonadotrophin.**

The **HCG discovery began** when the good doctor made this shrewd observation...

> "...refusing to be side tracked by the all too facile interpretation of obesity, I have always held that overeating is the RESULT of the disorder, not it's CAUSE..."

The **HCG hormone** in your system, **safely causes the loss of weight** by activating your warehoused 'abnormal fat' back into circulation where it can be accessed.

Adding to the protocol, a **Caloric intake of only 500 Calories daily,** under a **strict but simple plan of eating,** results in our body consuming our 'abnormal warehoused fat,' to **make up the balance** of our **daily Caloric needs.**

> "This normally results in weight loss of about a pound a day on average."

If you **follow the plan** carefully, **as prescribed** by Dr. Simeons, **you can achieve:**

- **Excellent Appetite Control**
- **Weight Loss Averaging About a Pound a Day**
- **Elimination of Inches of 'Warehoused Fat'**
- **Beneficial Health Results as a Side Effect!**
- **Steady and Rapid Decline of Your Obesity.**

> "Thus it is possible to leave your 'good' fat untouched and burn up your 'bad' fat."

You Can Defeat & Control Obesity Forever with the 'HCG + 500 Calorie Protocol'

"...I kept an open mind, did everything as perfect as I could, and **experienced eye-popping results**, in less than **63 days... I lost 55 pounds.**"

"**You will see** if you follow the protocol... that **this is the real deal.**"

"I **saw the results** with the **HCG diet** and decided to try it. I continued my exercise program each day and **shocked my trainer** when the results came back."

"I look at this diet as **sort of a miracle.**"

Absolutely **nothing I've ever tried** has been this **effective** or this **easy. I lost 35 pounds** so easily I felt like I was somehow cheating..."

"I made **a believer** out of **my trainer.**"

"When **understood correctly**, this HCG program is **not a weight loss program**, rather it is a once and for all **'cure for obesity...'**"

"In my opinion, the **HCG assisted diet protocol** is a genuine **medical marvel!**"

"...I **lost 100 pounds** in about **90 days**
and am keeping it off...

"...my **blood pressure** in now about **120 over 66** consistently.

"...HCG is **not a drug**; rather it is a
natural human hormone that
our body **'knows' exactly** how to use..."

"Great program, **easy**, and **it works**."

"I **reached 165** and have kept it off...
am **eating** and **feeling great**!"

"...the **line out of the doctor's door should
be about 10 miles long**!

"As of my last lab test my **total cholesterol** was at **138**
and glucose **under 100**."

"If followed as **exactly** laid out it is one
of the **easiest diets ever**."

"...an implementation of 'natural'
ways to **cure obesity...**"

" ...if **Doctor Simeons** were alive today he **would love** this fresh and **simple presentation** of his concepts..."

"...gives you all of the **knowledge, tools, understanding and motivation** to leave behind the life of obesity **forever...**

"...a **remarkably simple** and straight forward guide to success.... really **you shouldn't fail** if you follow the plan and **use the tools in this tool kit**... a really fine job."

"...use **this book** and you will be enjoying **life** in the **healthy, nutritional way** that was originally intended!"

...incredibly **simple and easy** to use... the **'HCG Victory Tool Kit'** certainly lives up to it's name...

"...an implementation of 'natural' ways to **cure obesity...**"

...this is exactly what I needed... a must have tool for **maximizing your success** and minimizing the confusion...

"...this is the **greatest HCG book** out there...

HCG VICTORY TOOL KIT

> *If some way...can be found*
> *to cope effectively with this*
> *universal problem*
> *of modern civilized man,*
> *our world will be a happier*
> *place for countless*
> *fellow men and women."*
>
> Dr. A. T. W. Simeons

Defeat OBESITY...Forever!

The HCG Assisted 500 Calorie Weight Loss Cure

HCG Victory Tool Kit

'You Can Defeat & Control Your Obesity...Forever!'

by James Walker

Printed in the United States of America

ISBN 978-0-9800641-7-9

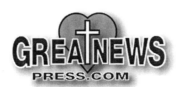

www.greatnewspress.com

Inspirational Books
Diet. Health & Nutrition

Introduction:

CONTENTS OVERVIEW

Section One:
'You Have
Chosen Wisely.'

Section One: 'You Have Chosen Wisely.'   Pages 17 - 28

You are reading it now. It is a welcome and introduction as well as an orientation and overview to the 'HCG Victory Tool Kit' and it's contents. Also you will find some case histories and testimonials from HCG alumni.

Section Two:
'Breaking the
Code'

Section Two: 'Breaking the Code.'   Pages 29 - 36

You will find a brief background of the nature of obesity and how it works, complete with flow charts and illustrations.

Also an overview of HCG + 500 Calorie Diet program and some guidelines for correctly, safely and successfully participating in it.

Section Three:
'Your Plan
for Victory!'

Health concerns and the impact of HCG on some of the more common pre-existing medical situations from Dr. Simeons experiences.

Section Three: 'Your Plan for Victory'   Pages 37 - 44

Specifics and a step by step guide where the 'rubber meets the road.' Follow the plan and you will be victorious.

Section Four:
'Tools for Victory.'

Section Four: 'Tools for Victory.'   Pages 45 - 98

Streamlined 'Food Tables' on the 4 food groups. Forms to plan your meals and track your progress. Sample menu plans and record keeping.

Section Five:
'Listen to the
Good Doctor.'

Section Five: 'LIsten to the Good Doctor.'   Pages 99 - 164

Re-formatted and polished up to improve readability and organization, the complete manuscript is reproduced here. Contains a glossary of terms and other references. For those of you that want the 'rest of the story.'

Section Six: 'A Tangled Web... Untangled.'   Pages 165 - 170

Web resources and additional helps. Books and web sites.

Section Six:
'A Tangled Web...
Untangled.'

Section Seven: 'Your Next Step.'   Pages 171 - 199

How to transition from the HCG assisted 500 Calorie Phase to setting your new body 'weight point' and returning to earth and leaving the 'fat' behind. 'No Sugar/No Starch' approved food tables and guidelines for success.

Section Seven:
'Your Next Step'

A GreatNewsPress.com catalog of additional books in this 'Victory' series and other inspirational books.

Introduction:

CONTENTS Detail

Introduction:

CONTENTS Detail

Introduction:

CONTENTS Detail

Section Seven:

'Taking the Next Step.'

Dedication:

Dr. A.T.W. Simeons

"The 'Einstein' of obesity."

I never met Dr. Simeons, or had even heard of his work while he was living, but I can tell from studying his writings, that I would have liked him a lot.

He strikes me as a dedicated, humble and unpretentious man, who had a genuine concern for the less fortunate. Through his medical research and study, he spent his life helping people. No baloney... just results.

I for one, am grateful. He was a good man. A 'cut to the chase' kind of guy with common sense. We need more like him. In his matter of fact way he understood the impact and accepted the irony of solving a less glamourous problem when he wistfully wrote the following...

"The problems of obesity are perhaps not so dramatic as the problems of cancer, or polio, but they often cause life long suffering."

"You can read Dr. Simeons manuscript detailing his discovery in his own words in Section 5."

He knew he would be ignored, and yet he did all the unglamorous, painstaking work anyway. He was doing it for you and for me, and the untold numbers of people whose lives have been altered for the better over the years, because of his work.

Please read about the 'Einstein of obesity.' Here is a very brief summary of his life.

Dr. Simeons was born in London and graduated in medicine (summa cum laude) at the University of Heidelberg. He completed post-graduate studies in Germany and Switzerland he was appointed to a large surgical hospital near Dresden.

Eventually he became engrossed in the study of tropical diseases, 'malaria' in particular and that led him to join the School of Tropical Medicine in Hamburg.

Following two years of work in Africa, he went to India in1931. He found himself so fascinated by the country and its health problems that he stayed for eighteen years.

He discovered the use of injectable 'atebrin' for malaria and was awarded a Red Cross Order of Merit. He developed a new method of 'staining' malaria parasites to identify them, that is still used even today, known as 'Simeons' stain.'

"... founding a model 'leper colony' which is now an all-India center."

During World War II, he held several important Government posts in India, conducting extensive research on bubonic plague and leprosy control, and founding a model 'leper colony' which is now an all-India center. During this time his interest in psychosomatic diseases began to develop.

He set up in private practice in Bombay for a time and then, with his wife and three sons, moved to Rome in 1949. Working on psychosomatic disorders, at the Salvator Mundi International Hospital.

Dr. Simeons is the author of several medical books also contributing to many scientific publications and journals.

His life ended in 1970. He is buried in the Cimeterio Accatolico in Rome, Italy.

Introduction:　FOREWORD to this 'TOOL KIT'

"This book discusses a new interpretation of the nature of obesity..."

What's it All About?

Here's what the good doctor had to say on the subject many years ago.*
I think it still rings true and clear...across the ages.

"This book discusses a **new interpretation** of the nature of obesity, and while it does not advocate another fancy slimming diet it does describe **a method of treatment** which has grown out of theoretical considerations based on clinical observation."

"What I have to say is an essence of views distilled out of forty years of grappling with the **fundamental problems of obesity**, its causes, its symptoms, and its very nature. In these many years of specialized work thousands of cases have passed through my hands and were carefully studied."

"...an essence of views distilled out of forty years of grappling with the fundamental problems of obesity, its causes, its symptoms, and its very nature."

"Refusing to be side-tracked by an all **too facile interpretation of obesity**, I have always held that overeating is the **result** of the disorder, **not its cause**, and that we can make little headway until we can build for ourselves some sort of theoretical structure with which to **explain the condition**."

"With mounting experience, more and more facts seemed to fit snugly into **the new framework**, and when then a **treatment based on such speculations** showed **consistently satisfactory results**, I was sure that some practical **advance** had been made, regardless of whether the theoretical interpretation of these results is correct."

"To make the text **more readable** I shall be **unashamedly authoritative** and avoid all the hedging and tentativeness with which it is customary to express new scientific concepts...**The expert** will grumble about long-windedness while **the lay-reader** may occasionally have to look up an unfamiliar word in the **glossary** provided."

"To make the text more readable I shall be unashamedly authoritative and avoid all the hedging and tentativeness..."

"In dealing with **a disorder** in which **the patient** must take an **active** part in the **treatment**, it is, I believe, **essential** that he or she have an **understanding** of **what** is being done and **why**.

Only then can there be **intelligent cooperation** between **physician** and **patient**."

This 'HCG Victory Tool Kit' is dedicated to the spirit of cooperation, between an enlightened doctor, and an understanding, comprehending, and focused patient, to achieve the cure of obesity...as espoused by Doctor Simeons.

Here's to your success.

JW　:]

*Excerpts from the 'Foreword' of Dr. Simeons manuscript

Introduction:

Let's Keep it as Simple as Possible.

What Time is It?

Did you hear about the person who was late for a meeting and didn't know the correct time? So they asked someone the time, and that person began to tell them how to build a clock! There are so many weight loss 'experts' out there, with lots to say... it's confusing!

Sometimes it seems to me it is confusing by design. If they made it simple and easy to understand... you wouldn't need them. Let's turn back the clock and **simplify**.

Keeping it Simple.

The objective of the **HCG Victory Tool Kit** and my purpose in putting it together is to **simplify** the whole thing. I am not a fitness guru, a nutrition expert or a doctor.

I am **not a salesman** for HCG.

What I am is a person, not much different than you, who was tired of the obesity battle and **frustrated** with all of the **extra fat** I was 'warehousing.'

I am just an average satisfied customer who is very excited about the potential of this HCG breakthrough. I want to **share** it with as many people as I can as fast as I can.

Like Dr. Simeons says "...the problems of obesity are not so dramatic as the problems of cancer or polio, but they often cause life long suffering." If you knew a cure for cancer that really worked and worked for everyone, could you keep it a secret?

As Simple as 1... 2... 3.

The **HCG Victory Tool Kit** is streamlined and simplified. It is easier not harder. It is not an exhaustive nutrition or food encyclopedia. As old Einstein said, "... the solution should be no more difficult than it needs to be..."

Step 1

The first step is to understand and carry out the **HCG + 500 Calorie** part of the plan. the beginning sections address that process in detail. You will also find **an overview** of the entire HCG plan. Understanding the process is **a key to success**.

You have in this **'Tool Kit'** an explanation of the **concept** and the **tools**, **tips** and **record** keeping **forms** you need to be **victorious**. A special **bonus** is a copy of Dr. Simeon's original manuscript, presented in **a fresh form**, that is **easy** to reference and read. So you can check the doctor's own words. Interesting stuff.

Everything you need to **be successful** with **HCG,** is contained in **Sections 1-6.**

They contain many **Caloric food tables** of common foods in the 4 food groups, that are readily available, day in and day out, for planning your meals while on HCG. As well as many other helpful tips and guides and basic recipes and preparation tips. The focus is on the foods **you can eat** not the ones you can't.

Step 2

The second step, **in Section Seven** shows you how to turn the corner, enter the **'No Sugar No-Starch Zone'** and set your body's natural weight management system. It is a critical key to **keeping the weight off for good** and moving forward.

"There are so many weight loss 'experts' out there with lots to say... it's confusing."

"If you knew a cure for cancer that really worked and worked for everyone, could you keep it a secret?"

Introduction: **Let's Keep it as Simple as Possible.**

Step 3

Recipes and tips for maintaining your new body and healthy eating lifestyle is the subject of the companion volume 'Recipes for Victory.' See page 197.

This is a **dynamic** addition that will continue to grow and evolve over time as new and better recipes are uncovered and contributed. Experiment. Invent your own recipes and share them. Plan to enjoy your new life and the taste of weight loss success!

Other Helpful Tools Coming Soon.

The all new 'HCG Victory Planner' will be available soon. The planner contains a series of **already prepared** menu plans for both the 'HCG + 500 Calorie' phase and the 'No Sugar-No Starch ZONE.** The prepared 7 day menu plans are available in 1200 to 2500 Daily Calorie targets in 100 Calorie increments! **A real time saver.**

"One of the most amazing things about this HCG plan is that it works so quickly."

Plus you will find plenty of blank 5 day and 7 day menu planners and other record keeping helps and tips. **Check our website: www.HCGVictoryToolKit.com**

'Poof' It Works Like Magic.

One of the most **amazing** things about this HCG plan is that it **works so quickly**.

Reviewing my own records, I lowered my weight by **22.5 pounds**, my **blood sugar** by **139 points**, without medication... in the **first week**. Others have reported similar results some even better. Dr. Simeons claim of 'on average loss of about a pound a day,' does hold true, repeatedly.

Women typically don't lose as fast or as much daily as men, but reach their goals, just the same. Women have other biological influences at work, as well as, the use of oils and cosmetics. Not to mention massages, manicures and pedicures!

You will experience plateaus and temporary set backs, but the pay off is there if you persevere. You will be **amazed** at your final result. We **all are amazed** at the end!

Lose it Sooner... Not Later.

Rapid feedback is one of the perks and helps **to keep you motivated**.

"I don't walk around hollow eyed and hungry."

When I reviewed my first week results, I knew that **I had found the answer** I had been looking for. Here was something that worked exactly like it was supposed to.

It was **easy to stay motivated** and to pay the 'price' because I could sense that the reward was worth it. I was right. I lost **55** pounds in **63 days** and I found a permanent solution. I had the magic bullet. Obesity in my life is now in the past. I am free from the chains of obesity and the multiple prescriptions. My blood sugar is now normal.

Today I **easily maintain** my weight, I eat better than I ever have, and I eat loads of nutritious, delicious and healthy foods, I don't walk around hollow eyed and hungry.

I am FREE.

You will be too. Just **go for it!**

Section One:

'You Have Chosen Wisely.'

> *"The problems of obesity are perhaps not so dramatic as the problems of cancer, or polio, but they often cause life long suffering."*
>
> Dr. A.T.W. Simeons

Defeat OBESITY...Forever!

The HCG Assisted 500 Calorie Weight Loss Cure

Section One: **'You Have Chosen Wisely'**

"You have chosen to break free..."

"You are on the road to increasing vitality and health."

"HCG is amazing and it works."

Welcome and Congratulations!

Want to **defeat and control obesity** forever? You have found the genuine answer.

One of my favorite 'Indiana Jones' movies has a scene where Indy has to choose a drinking cup which he will dip into the eternal spring to drink the miraculous elixir of health and life. He passes over many fancy and gilded cups and settles on a very plain, ordinary and unpretentious one. He dips it and drinks. The guardian of the cups watches carefully and then quietly declares, "You have chosen wisely."

You have also 'chosen wisely.' You have chosen to break free from the chains of obesity and creeping health concerns. I welcome you and congratulate you sincerely with all my heart. Thank you for choosing the **HCG Victory Tool Kit**.

Victory is possible. A great and momentous **changed life** is before you.

Let me say it again... **"You... have chosen wisely!"**

A Medical Marvel.

Many others have gone before you, not only succeeding in getting down to their **weight goals** but continuing to **maintain** their chosen weight. You can lose the pounds and inches you want to lose and keep the body you want to have. Out the window with the pills and back on the road to **increasing vitality and health.**

The Good Doctor.

Dr. Simeons **dedicated his life** for over 40 years to grappling with a very unglamorous subject... obesity. What he discovered is, in my opinion, a complete medical marvel. I am **still amazed**, as are many, many others who are 'fat free' at last.

At almost 65 years of age, the last 20 spent struggling with obesity, and trying everything to defeat it, while my health and life expectancy slowly dwindled, I finally found **the answer.** You are at the gateway, that I passed through to victory.

Dr A.T.W. Simeons is like that simple plain, unpretentious and humble cup that Indy chose. He is the vehicle... the elixir is **Human Chorionic Gonadotrophin** which we shall simply call **HCG** from this point forward. Difficult to pronounce and not exactly accurately named. It doesn't matter if you can say it... HCG is amazing and it works.

The 'HCG Victory Tool Kit.'

Here's what this **'Tool Kit'** concept is all about. Showing you how to succeed as simply and easily as possible, and giving you the tools you need, to victoriously complete the **500 Calorie HCG assisted** phase of Dr. Simeons weight loss cure.

Every section is streamlined to **focus** on what **you must do** and what **you can eat** and the protocol for succeeding. I have included a straightforward and **simple explanation** of everything you need, and if you want to go deeper, you will find Dr. Simeon's manuscript also included in **Section Five: 'Listen to the Good Doctor.'** Even that manuscript has been polished up and presented in an **easier to read** format, with important **concepts** highlighted, a few **charts** and a **table of contents**.

Take a few minutes on the following pages to read some **HCG alumni success stories**. As incredible as it sounds they are pretty typical of the HCG experience.

HCG ALUMNI

CASE HISTORIES

HCG ALUMNI · CASE HISTRIES

ISBN 978-0-9800641-7-9

Section One: **HCG Alumni Case Histories**

HCG Alumni Case History:

James

Age: 64

"...a genuine medical marvel!"

"...inspired me to try to help as many people as possible find the answer to their weight loss dreams by writing and publishing this 'HCG Victory Tool Kit."

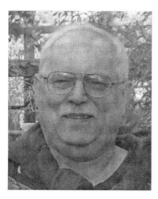

BEFORE HCG:

Weight: 247
Waist size: 44

Weight Related Medical Concerns:
Weight, blood sugar, blood pressure, cholesterol, RX side effects, costs.

Number of RX: 4-5
RX Cost: $750 Mo.

AFTER HCG:

Weight: 192
Waist size: 36

Medical Concerns:

NONE

Number of RX: 0
RX Cost: $0 Mo.

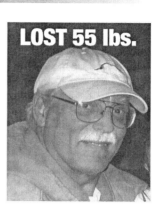

LOST 55 lbs.

This is **my story** and also **what inspired me** to create this **HCG Victory Tool Kit.**

Struggling with my weight for about the last **20 years**, I was **unhappy and unhealthy** plus suffering from the **side effects** of the prescriptions I was taking daily. A big expense, plus **I was going nowhere fast**, in the lifestyle area.

Over the years, I have **tried many different approaches** to losing weight with little success. Working out 7 days a week didn't lose the fat... strict dieting didn't lose the fat... nothing was removing the fat from the **areas I was trying to remove it from... nothing would last**!

I did everything I was asked to do by the 'big box' establishment doctors and their 'pill pushing' approach to medicine. Not only was it **not very effective** with many **undesirable side effects**, I ended up with undiagnosed pneumonia and **almost died**. I didn't want to spend **the rest of my life** in and out of doctors offices.

I couldn't figure out what was going on. My **health** was **slowly deteriorating**.

I came to an **'evolution of decision,'** it was time to try something different!

Seeking answers outside of the mainstream medical 'herd,' I located an 'enlightened' doctor with **fresh new ideas**. She suggested the **HCG 500 Calorie diet**.

Of course **I thought she meant** 500 Calories PER MEAL! Wow. But, I kept an **open mind**, did everything as perfect as I could, and experienced **eye-popping results**. I lost **over 20 pounds** in the **first week**! At that point I began to think... ' this is the **real deal...**' and so I focused on doing everything as instructed... I was right...in **63 days I lost 55 pounds**.

I have since **shared the knowledge** with the many people who noticed the changes in me and many of them have done the same.

In my opinion, the **HCG assisted diet protocol** is a **genuine medical marvel**!

You will see if you **follow the protocol**... that this is **the 'real deal.'**

That is what **inspired me** to try to help as many people as possible find the answer to their weight loss dreams by writing and publishing this **'HCG Victory Tool Kit.'**

Find yourself an **enlightened doctor** use **certified HCG** supplied by a **legitimate pharmacy** and **use all of the tools** and **instructions** in this guide... and **you will win** your battle with obesity... **just like I did**.

Section One: **HCG Alumni Case Histories**

HCG Alumni
Case History:

Linda

Age: 59

"I look at this
diet as a
sort of
a miracle!"

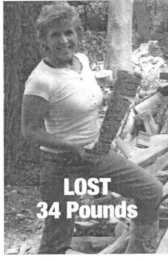

LOST
34 Pounds

AFTER HCG:

Weight: 126

Weight Related
Medical Concerns:

NONE
Number of RX: 0
RX Cost: $0 Mo.

I am extremely serious about being as healthy as possible for my age. **I worked hard** at exercise, eating right, and dieting, for years and virtually **made no progress**.

I wanted off of my medications.

Nothing was working for me to accomplish my weight loss goals or getting my **blood pressure** down, without the meds.

I **saw the results** with the HCG diet and decided to try it. I continued my exercise program each day and **shocked my trainer** when the results came back. He thought I would lose muscle mass and bone density and not lose that much fat. I went **up in muscle mass and bone density** and **down in fat percentage**, drastically. I **made a believer** out of him.

Absolutely **nothing I've ever tried** has been this **effective** or this **easy**. I **felt like I was cheating** the diet system somehow.

I look at this diet as **sort of a miracle**.

BEFORE HCG:

Weight: 160

Weight Related
Medical Concerns:

Weight, blood pressure, RX side effects & costs.

Number of RX: 1-2
RX Cost: $250 Mo.

HCG Alumni
Case History:

Jim

Age 54

"...the line out of
the doctors door
should be
ten miles long."

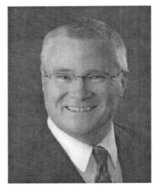

BEFORE HCG:	**AFTER HCG:**
Weight: 212	**Weight: 165**
Waist size: 36	**Waist size: 32**
Weight Related Medical Concerns:	Weight Related Medical Concerns:
NONE	NONE
Number of RX:	Number of RX:
RX Cost:	RX Cost:

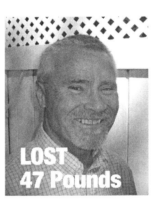

LOST
47 Pounds

Although I didn't have any **weight related health problems**, I knew if I didn't win my 30 year '**battle of the bulge**,' I could be at risk as I got older.

One benefit was, although I had **no high blood pressure** concerns, my **blood pressure went way down** even though it was not too high before.

I experienced **no problems** with my allergy medicine and no changes were needed. I really **wanted to lose weight and I did**.

This is a **great program**, **easy**, and it **works**. The line out of the doctors door should be about 10 miles long. I reached 165 and **have kept it off** and I am **eating great and feeling great!**

Section One: **Case Histories: Before & After**

HCG Alumni Case History:

Dave

Age 60

"I was sick and tired of being sick and tired!"

"...understood correctly the HCG program is not a 'weight loss' program... rather it is a once and for all cure for obesity..."

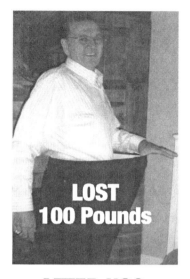

LOST 100 Pounds

AFTER HCG:

Weight: 200
Waist size: 36

Medical Concerns:

NONE

Number of RX: 0
RX Cost: $0 Mo.

I wanted to lose weight primarily for health reasons and also, just the embarrassment and inconvenience of being obese. When you're carrying around an **"extra' 100 pounds**, it's **disgusting** to realize that you can't even do something as simple as "tying your shoe" without nearly passing out. I could **not** get a good night's **sleep** without using a machine to help me breathe! Basically, I was 'Sick and Tired of being Sick and Tired' and I knew it was **all because of my weight!**

The **HCG program** has been well researched and is an attempt to cure obesity, not just manage it. It's all based on research and is an implementation of the **'natural' ways** to cure obesity, by first detoxifying our body, of the pesticides and preservatives, that we find in most of our food. HCG is not a drug... it is **a natural human hormone** that our body 'knows' how to use.

It is quite simple, and surprisingly, **very satisfying**.

No 'Killer Hunger Pains' in the process. If followed as exactly laid out, it is **one of the easiest diets ever**.

It's like a 'walk in the park' compared to some programs. The loss of, anywhere from a **one half to a full pound per DAY**, yes... per day, is the consistent reward and immediate satisfaction that helps you maintain the mental determination to continue the **HCG + 500 Calorie** phase of the process, because **you realize it is working** and it's a temporary situation that pays off.

BEFORE HCG:

Weight: 300
Waist size: 46

Medical Concerns:
Weight, blood pressure, cholesterol & sleeping problems.

Number of RX: 2-3
RX Cost: $200 Mo.
$3000. Sleep Aid

I'm not finished... but have only just begun **a whole new life** and world of living in the **nutritional trim and fit way** that my body was originally designed for! That's the wonderful part... knowing that **I never have to go back** to my old body.

When understood correctly, this HCG program is not a weight loss program, rather it is a once and for all **'cure for obesity'** that gives you all of the knowledge, tools, understanding and motivation to leave behind the life of obesity **forever** and the ability to move forward enjoying life in the **healthy, nutritional way** that life was originally intended to be!

I was able to have some postponed, needed surgeries, after losing all of the weight.

My **doctors were impressed** with all of my pre-op test results. All of my poor health conditions had made me a poor candidate for surgery, prior to completing my HCG obesity cure! **I was then able to successfully complete the surgeries.**

I feel like a **'new person,'** just **starting my great adventure** of good, nutritional eating and enjoyment for the **rest of my life**!

Section One: Write Your Success Story Here!

Case History:

HCG Alumni

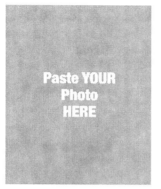

BEFORE HCG:

Weight:
Waist:

Medical Concerns:

Number of RX:
RX Cost:

AFTER HCG:

Weight:
Waist:

Medical Concerns:

Number of RX:
RX Cost:

Your Story:

Case History:

HCG Alumni

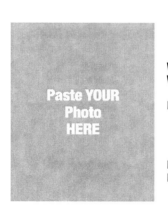

BEFORE HCG:

Weight:
Waist:

Medical Concerns:

Number of RX:
RX Cost:

AFTER HCG:

Weight:
Waist:

Medical Concerns:

Number of RX:
RX Cost:

Your Story:

Section One: Write Your Success Story Here!

Case History:

HCG Alumni

Paste YOUR Photo HERE

BEFORE HCG:

Weight:
Waist:

Medical Concerns:

Number of RX:
RX Cost:

AFTER HCG:

Weight:
Waist:

Medical Concerns:

Number of RX:
RX Cost:

Paste YOUR Photo HERE

Your Story:

Case History:

HCG Alumni

Paste YOUR Photo HERE

BEFORE HCG:

Weight:
Waist:

Medical Concerns:

Number of RX:
RX Cost:

AFTER HCG:

Weight:
Waist:

Medical Concerns:

Number of RX:
RX Cost:

Paste YOUR Photo HERE

Your Story:

Section Two:

'Breaking the Code'

> *"How many promising careers have been ruined by excessive fat; how many lives have been shortened?"*
>
> *Dr. A.T.W. Simeons*

Defeat OBESITY...Forever!

The HCG Assisted 500 Calorie Weight Loss Cure

ISBN 978-0-9800641-7-9

Section Two: **'Breaking the Code'**

"Refusing to be side-tracked by an all too facile interpretation of obesity, I have always held that overeating is the result of the disorder, not its cause..."

"...the patient must take an active part in the treatment..."

"...it is, I believe, essential that he or she have an understanding of what is being done and why..."

Winning the Battle of the 'Bulge.'

In **every great conflict** there are advances and retreats and a necessary price to pay. The nagging question is always... **"Was it worth the cost?"**

Sometimes great battles turn on the most unglamorous discovery made by some **humble, hard working** individual or group. Often the impact of that discovery far out weighs the recognition it receives and those who pioneered it are pushed aside and forgotten. Even more tragic is a **lack of understanding**, by those in the mainstream, of the potential significance of a breakthrough, and so it is under utilized.

Dr. Simeons discovery pertaining to the use of an **HCG + 500 Calorie** protocol for treating obesity may be one of those discoveries. You and I are the lucky ones. Because of his work, we at last, have the opportunity to **be victorious** over obesity.

When I first discovered this 'HCG thingy' as I first referenced it, and the amazing way it worked, two questions came to mind. **'Why had I not heard of it before?'** which I think, we just answered, and **'Was it worth the cost?'**

Worth the Cost?

There is always **a price to pay**. Here is how I look at the cost issue.

In my case, I could **invest** some money and 'buy' **my life** back and reverse my downward spiral of failing health and compromised lifestyle or... I could continue to **'rent' my life** from the 'big box' doctors and RX companies. I am **not sorry** in any way for my choice to break free. Now I really am free from obesity forever, and I feel great. I am looking forward to my 'sunset' years with **confidence and hope**.

Everyone's **cost will vary**, depending on the pounds and inches you need to lose and your current **medical conditions** and of course your **overall health** lifestyle.

Was it worth the cost? Yes! Every penny. I am **saving $500 to $750** per month, that I was spending on prescriptions, and I am **eating better**, healthier and more than I ever have in my entire life. **Yet my weight stays right where I want it**. I love it.

How is this Possible?

Because the 'old doctor' **cracked the code of obesity** and spent over 40 years of his life perfecting a way to **teach** and treat others. Many long hours, many trials and errors figuring out the pieces of the puzzle. A rather unglamorous, quiet and unassuming work.

In his manuscript (**Section Five: 'Listen to the Good Doctor'**) he mentions other medical professionals coming from around the world to study his work, but **not devoting the time** and consideration to make proper use of his discoveries. Must have been so frustrating for him, as he was an **unselfish and dedicated** man.

But **he persevered**, and now **we can reap the benefits**.

Thank you, Dr. Simeons.

Know the Enemy: Three Kinds of Fat.

Before you can fully buy into this whole **HCG + 500 Calorie** concept, you need a brief background on what makes us obese... that would be 'fat.' Here's a few explanations from Dr. Simeons on the subject, that will **help you understand**, how this whole protocol works.

"In the human body we can distinguish three kinds of fat."

"In the **human body** we can distinguish **three kinds of fat**.

The **first** is the **structural fat** which fills the gaps between various organs, a sort of packing material. Structural fat also performs such important functions as bedding the kidneys in soft elastic tissue, protecting the coronary arteries and keeping the skin smooth and taut. It also provides the springy cushion of hard fat under the bones of the feet, without which we would be unable to walk.

A **second type of fat** is a **normal reserve of fuel** on which the body can freely draw when the nutritional income from the intestinal tract is insufficient to meet the demand. Such normal reserves are localized all over the body.

Fat is a substance which packs the **highest caloric value into the smallest space** so that normal reserves of fuel for muscular activity and the maintenance of body temperature can be most economically stored in this form.

Both these types of fat, **structural and reserve, are normal**, and even if the body stocks them to capacity this can never be called obesity.

But there is **a third type of fat which is entirely abnormal**.

It is the accumulation of such fat, and of such fat only, from which the over weight patient suffers. This **abnormal fat** is also a **potential** reserve of fuel, but unlike the normal reserves **it is not available to the body** in a nutritional emergency.

It is, so to speak, **locked away in a fixed deposit** and is not kept in a current account as are the normal reserves."

"Only then can there be intelligent cooperation between physician and patient."

OK. Does that make sense? Some fat is needed, some fat is good and is like a 'current account' or as we would say a 'checking account.' We make deposits into this reserve for current and possible short term shortages. A 'put and take' arrangement. I like to think in terms of **'dynamic'** fat as opposed to **'static'** fat.

The third kind of fat, **'static fat'**... is our real enemy. This fat is **warehoused** all over our body, seen and unseen, it is **the root cause of our obesity**. This excess fat warehoused in our body, is **normally unavailable** for our Caloric needs. Remember that term, **'warehouse fat,'** as we will refer to it again.

Understanding where the **'bad fat'** comes from, our objective now becomes **how to eliminate and control it**. Once again, Dr. Simeons has the answer.

What Mechanism Controls Our 'Static' Fat?

"Many obese patients actually gain weight on a diet which is calorically deficient for their basic needs."

After many tests and trials and following up on many promising theories Dr. Simeons hit upon **the answer at last**.

> "The **diencephalon** is the part from which the **central nervous system** controls **all the automatic animal functions of the body,** such as breathing, the heart beat, digestion, sleep, sex, the urinary system, the autonomous or vegetative nervous system and via the pituitary the whole interplay of the endocrine glands.

> It was therefore **not unreasonable to suppose** that the complex operation of storing and issuing fuel to the body might also be **controlled by the diencephalon**."

The what? Maybe I was absent that day in health class. I thought to myself... 'what in the world is a diencephalon?' I found out. It is just another word for hypothalamus. Boy that helps a lot doesn't it?

The Diencephalon or Hypothalamus.

"There must thus be some other mechanism at work."

It is a part of the brain about the size of a walnut in an adult. It is an amazing and mysterious central control system that monitors and regulates all of the other glands in the body, thus it controls all autonomic functions. Those things that take place without a conscious thought, breathing, thirst, hunger... wait a minute... hunger? Another piece to the puzzle. Dr. Simeons wondered, 'Could it be that **this area of the brain** also controls the operation of storing and issuing fuel in the form of fat to the body...?'

> "Assuming that in man such **a center controlling the movement of fat** does exist, its function would have to be much like that of a bank. When the body assimilates from the intestinal tract more fuel than it needs at the moment, this **surplus is deposited** in what may be compared with a 'current account.' (Note: he is referring to a 'checking account')

> Out of this account it can always be withdrawn as required. All normal fat reserves are in such a current account, and **it is probable** that a **diencephalic center** manages the deposits and withdrawals."

He goes on to theorize.

"The onset of obesity dates from the moment the diencephalon adopts this labor-saving ruse."

> "...a point may be reached which goes beyond the diencephalon's banking capacity. Just as a banker might suggest to a wealthy client that instead of accumulating a large and unmanageable current account he should invest his surplus capital, **the body appears to establish a fixed deposit** into which all surplus funds go but from which they can **no longer be withdrawn** by the procedure used in a 'current account.' In this way the diencephalic **'fat-bank'** frees itself from all work which goes beyond its normal banking capacity.

> The onset of obesity dates from the moment the diencephalon adopts this labor-saving ruse. Once a fixed deposit has been established the normal fat reserves are held at a minimum, while **every available surplus is locked away in the fixed deposit** and is therefore taken **out of normal circulation**."

'Breaking the Code'

A Brilliant Discovery.

Why Dr. Simeons didn't receive a Nobel Prize for his work is hard to fathom.

He has a lot more to say about the nature of obesity and several medical facets of it's nature, but we are just looking at the essence of his discovery and that is all we need to do at this point. If you want all of the details, read **Section Five: 'Listen to the Good Doctor.'** It really is interesting reading.

Where the 'Rubber Meets the Road.'

So let's review what we have covered so far.

We have **good fat** and **bad fat**. The bad fat is 'static' or warehouse fat. **The storage and movement of fat** in our bodies is controlled by that part of **our brain** called the **hypothalamus.** We all have a fat bank or **'fat warehouse.'** and when it begins, **obesity soon follows**, as the **'static fat'** goes in and stays there **unused.**

The **hypothalamus** of course is the **author and manager** of that warehouse.

So how can this help us triumph over our obesity? Let's look at what the doctor did.

"So how can we triumph over our obesity?"

> "...I remembered **a rather curious observation** made many years ago in India. At that time we knew very little about the function of the diencephalon..."

> ...giving the patients injections of a substance extracted from the urine of pregnant women... the purified extract was accordingly called "Human Chorionic Gonadotrophin" whereby 'chorionic' signifies that it is produced in the placenta and 'gonadotropin' that its action is sex gland directed.

> **Human Chorionic Gonadotrophin** which we shall henceforth simply call **HCG...** I tried to establish the smallest effective dose. In the course of this study three interesting things emerged.

> The first was that when fresh pregnancy-urine from the female ward was given in quantities of about 300 cc. by retention enema, as good results could be obtained as by injecting the pure substance.

> The second was that **small daily doses** appeared to be just as effective as much larger ones given twice a week.

"...the purified extract was accordingly called Human Chorionic Gonadotrophin"

> Thirdly, and that is **the observation that concerns us here**, when such patients were given small daily doses **they seemed to lose their ravenous appetite** though they **neither gained nor lost weight. Strangely enough however, their shape did change.** Though they **were not restricted in diet**, there was **a distinct decrease** in the circumference of their hips."

Section Two: **'Breaking the Code'**

Another **piece of the puzzle** identified. Further studies quantified this discovery.

> "Remembering this, it occurred to me that the change in shape could **only be explained by a movement of fat away from abnormal deposits** on the hips, and if that were so **there was just a chance** that while such fat was in transition it might be **available to the body as fuel**...

"...the change in shape could only be explained by a movement of fat away from abnormal deposits... "

> ... I found that as long as such patients were given **small daily doses of HCG** they could **comfortably** go about their usual occupations on a diet of only **500 Calories daily** and **lose an average of about one pound per day**.

> It was also perfectly evident that **only abnormal fat was being consumed**, as there were no signs of any depletion of normal fat. Their skin remained fresh and turgid, and gradually **their figures became entirely normal, nor did the daily administration of HCG appear to have any side-effects other than beneficial**.

> From this point it was a small step to try the same method in all other forms of obesity. It took a few hundred cases **to establish beyond reasonable doubt** that **the mechanism operates in exactly the same way** and seemingly **without exception** in every case of obesity.

> I found that, though most patients were treated in the outpatient department, gross dietary errors rarely occurred. On the contrary, most patients complained that **the two meals of 250 Calories** each were more than they could manage, as they continually **had a feeling of just having had a large meal**."

Rejoice! The 'Obesity' Code is Broken.

Ding Dong! The witch is dead.

There you have it. The reader's digest version of Dr. Simeon's amazing discovery and a brief preview of **how it works**. As Albert Einstein said, 'The solution when found... will be simple.' Not only is it **simple** when found, **it works**!

"...nor did the daily administration of HCG appear to have any side-effects other than beneficial."

In my opinion, Dr. Simeons is the 'Einstein' of obesity.

If you are like me you have tried lots of other treatments for your obesity, with varying success. This is different. Follow the protocol, trust the 'old doctor' and win big.

You are **no different** than any other human on the planet, thus I believe the **'HCG + 500 Calorie'** protocol will work for you, just like **it has for many, many others**.

In the **next section** we will lay out your plan for **a permanent victory** in greater detail, as well as point out a few **cautions and advisories** from Dr. Simeons.

We will also cover the **equipment** you will need, and **share some ideas** to help you get the most out of your HCG experience.

Section Three:

'Your Plan for Victory.'

> *"No end of injustice is done to obese patients by accusing them of compulsive eating..."*
>
> Dr. A.T.W. Simeons

Defeat OBESITY...Forever!

The HCG Assisted 500 Calorie Weight Loss Cure

ISBN 978-0-9800641-7-9

Section Three: **'Your Plan for Victory'**

Victory Over Obesity!

You should now be starting to realize that **Dr. Simeons research** and **testing** has **unlocked an incredible technique**, harnessing the body's **natural processes**, to **eliminate** and **control** abnormal or 'warehouse fat.'

Let's **review** what we know so far about the problem of 'warehouse' or static fat and what we can do about it. Then we will **outline the exact procedure** to follow.

We have **three kinds of fat**:

> 1) **'structural fat'** (good and necessary)
> 2) **'dynamic fat'** (our reserve fat fuel 'checking account')
> 3) **'static fat'** (bad fat and the source of our obesity, our 'fat warehouse')

The 'static fat' is just going to sit in our body's warehouse forever. It is **dead weight**. We must do something about it specifically or we cannot win the battle.

Our brain's **diencephalon** or **hypothalamus** monitors and controls the movement of fat in our body and is responsible for the **excess fat warehousing** function.

HCG is the mercifully short acronym for **Human Chorionic Gonadotrophin.**

HCG is derived from the urine of pregnant women and plays **a key nutritional role** for anyone, male or female, when given in small regular doses in concert with the 500 Calorie structured daily food consumption.

This combination of **HCG + 500 Calories** produces several very desirable effects.

Activation by the HCG of the **abnormal fat back into circulation,** where it is consumed by the body at the rate of about **a pound a day on average. Appetite control** with the **consumption of only 500 Calories**, and **weight and inches eliminated** due to the **steady and rapid consumption of the 'warehouse fat.'**

Thus it is possible to leave the **good fat** untouched and **burn up the bad fat**.

Dr. Simeons to the Rescue... again!

What is left for us to do is figure out **exactly what kinds of foods** to use to make up our **500 Calorie daily menu**. Good old Doctor Simeons has already done that and tested and perfected the proper meal plans for us. **Specific Food Tables** by group are in **Section Four: 'Your Tools for Victory'** along with other valuable **references** and all the **food charts, menu planners** and **record keeping tools**.

Needles are Not Needed.

If you have read ahead in Dr. Simeon's manuscript you might have noticed words like 'injection' and other references to needles and shots. You can relax, **no shots are necessary** to successfully complete the 500 Calorie HCG assisted weight loss cure. The 'sublingual' method is the answer. That's doctor talk for put it under your tongue and absorb it. It is easy to do in minutes and taste free. The HCG we have now is so pure and potent that shots are not required. Did somebody say 'whew?' Next is Dr. Simeons outline of your plan for victory. More specifics in Section Four.

"...Dr. Simeons research and testing has unlocked an incredible technique..."

"Activation by the HCG of the abnormal fat back into circulation where it is consumed by the body at the rate of about a pound a day on average."

Section Three: **The 500 Calorie + HCG Diet**

Here is Dr. Simeons ORIGINAL 500 calorie diet plan.

Breakfast:

Tea or coffee in any quantity without sugar. Only one tablespoonful of milk allowed in 24 hours. Saccharin* or Stevia may be used.

Lunch:

Protein: 100 grams of veal, beef, chicken breast, fresh white fish, lobster, crab, or shrimp. All visible fat must be carefully removed before cooking, and the meat must be weighed raw. It must be boiled or grilled without additional fat. Salmon, eel, tuna, herring, dried or pickled fish are not allowed. The chicken breast must be removed from the bird.

Vegetable: One type of vegetable only to be chosen from the following: spinach, chard, chicory, beet-greens, green salad, tomatoes, celery, fennel, onions, red radishes, cucumbers, asparagus, cabbage.

Fruit: An apple, orange, or one-half grapefruit.

Breads: One breadstick (grissino) or one Melba toast.

Dinner:

Choose from the same four groups as lunch shown above BUT **avoid the same choice twice in a row**. i.e. if you have chicken for lunch then have a **different protein** choice for dinner.

Condiments & Seasonings:

The juice of one lemon daily is allowed for all purposes. Salt, pepper, vinegar, mustard powder, garlic, sweet basil, parsley, thyme, marjoram, etc., if they contain **NO SUGAR**, may be used for seasoning. **NO** oil, butter or dressing.

Drinks & Fluid Intake:

"...the patient should drink about 2 liters of these fluids per day."

Tea, coffee, plain water, or mineral water are the only drinks allowed, but they may be taken in any quantity and at all times. Remember **NO SUGAR**.

In fact, the patient should **drink about 2 liters** of these fluids per day. Many patients are afraid to drink so much because they fear that this may make them retain more water. This is a wrong notion as the body is more inclined to store water when the intake falls below its normal requirements.

The fruit or the breadstick may be eaten between meals instead of at lunch or dinner, but **not more than than four items**, one in each category listed, may be eaten at one meal. Remember to alternate your choices.

* See 'Sugars: Natural & Un-natural' in Section Four

Section Three: **The 500 Calorie + HCG Diet**

"This is a doctor directed treatment."

Digesting the Diet Plan.

Pardon the pun. Some comments are appropriate to illuminate the good doctor's original outline. Some of the measurements are metric, so let's look at that first.

100 grams of meat is **3.75** ounces **always weighed RAW**. No need to get a fancy scale. An inexpensive postal scale works just fine.

Note that there are **four food groups** listed for victory:

Group One:	**Proteins**
Group Two:	**Vegetables**
Group Three:	**Fruits**
Group Four:	**Starch (in the form of Bread)**

These groups are specifically outlined for you in **Section Four**. Be sure to **rotate your choices** so you are not eating the same thing twice in a row, for instance:

Lunch: chicken, lettuce, apple, Melba toast

Dinner: beef, fresh spinach, grapefruit, breadstick

"...use your common sense and find an enlightened doctor that treats you with respect."

Get the idea? Change is important. Stay true to the approved choices. Dr. Simeons spent over 40 years working this out, just **trust it**, fly straight and **you will win**.

Do Not Exceed 500 Calories per Day.

You will also find some **suggested menu plans** as well as a variety of **forms** for developing **your own menu plans** and tracking and **recording your progress** in **Section Four**.

A variety of **'sweeteners'** that are okay to use, are outlined there as well, and some helpful basic recipes.

A **liter** is about 34 ounces, so 2 liters a day equals 68 ounces. Bottled water is 12 to 20 ounces, a large paper cup of espresso (black) is about 20 ounces. It adds up fast. **Not** getting **enough liquid** can stall your progress, so be sure to do it right.

Check your spices and condiments very carefully, for any sugar, or oil ingredients.

Existing Health Concerns and Common Sense.

"...your health... ...ultimately it is your responsibility."

Many of the **side effects** of HCG are **beneficial** to your health and your body.

Please read Dr. Simeons cautions in his manuscript in Section Five: 'Listen to the Good Doctor' **(note pages 133-136)** and of course **discuss with your doctor** any concerns you may have. This is a physician directed treatment, use your common sense and find an **enlightened doctor** that treats you with respect. Take charge of your health and well being, ultimately you are your responsibility... not your doctors.

Obtain **your** complete **medical records** and keep it up to date by adding test results as they come up and anything else worthy of note. Always comes in handy.

Weighing in on Weighing In.

Not mentioned in Dr. Simeons description of the **500 Calorie + HCG** diet, are a couple of important procedures that we need to take a look at now.

One procedure, that many people find puzzling, is the practice of 'gorging' on as much fatty, high Calorie food you can get your hands on for a minimum of two days before you begin the 500 Calorie part of the HCG diet. Listen to the old doctor...

"...very hard to convince of the absolute necessity of gorging for at least two days..."

"...patients who have been struggling with diets for years and know how rapidly they gain if they let themselves go are very hard to convince of the **absolute necessity of gorging for at least two days**, and yet this must he **insisted upon categorically** if the further course of treatment is to run smoothly."

This is **not optional**. Sure you will gain a few pounds, but doing this like the doctor says is **critical to your success**. Need I say more?

The second thing not mentioned, but worth pointing out again, is something we are all curious about, and often relieved to discover. **Needles are not required.** You mix your HCG solution **five days at a time**, and then twice daily, place the prescribed amount of the clear, tasteless liquid under your tongue, (sublingual method) hold it for three minutes without swallowing. That's all there is to it.

Take a look at the big picture on the '**HCG Overview Flow Chart**' on **page 44**.

Staying the 'Course.'

One other important issue, that will come up sooner or later, is the '**HCG Immunity syndrome**' discussed at length in the doctor's manuscript.

"HCG today is much more potent and you may safely repeat the twenty day course..."

In Dr. Simeons day this was a major issue and a limiting factor in the duration of treatment. HCG today is much **more potent** and pure and you may safely repeat the twenty day 'course' as he calls it, up to 6 months (180 days) continuously, under the direction of your physician. This allows you to take maximum advantage of the 'self limiting' aspect of this protocol. When you have emptied your body of it's '**abnormal fat**' you will, of course, **stop losing pounds and inches**.

That's your sign... It's **time to move on** to the next stage.

So if you have more than 20 pounds to lose you can keep right on going. In addition, you can always return to the program any time in the future, if you feel you need a 'tune-up,' without any problem, and usually with even greater ease, since as an HCG alumnus, you know the system and how to manage the diet successfully.

Equip Yourself for Success.

You do need some equipment to correctly prepare, manage and track your success.

- A **scale** for weighing raw meat. An inexpensive postal scale works fine. Anything that will **accurately** measure 3.75 ounces (100 grams) Of course you must **practice good hygiene** when working with raw meat. Always wash your hands thoroughly (at least 30 seconds) with hot soapy water, **before and after** working with meat. Carefully wash

Section Three: **The 500 Calorie + HCG Diet**

"Yes, it is important to be as precise as possible."

all utensils as well. I used some of those small styrofoam trays to hold the raw meat while weighing it. Then simply **clean and disinfect** the tray for reuse.

Another tip is to do your meat in **batches**. Trim and weigh enough for a couple of days at a time. A bonus advantage is you can marinate your protein which adds flavor and appetite appeal. Remember you can use a wide array of seasonings, as long as they are FAT FREE, SUGAR FREE, and OIL FREE. Try cooking in batches, using a 'George Foreman Fat Free Grill,' your oven, or barbecue.

• 'George Foreman **Fat Free Grill**.' Or as George likes to say "...the Lean Mean Grillin' Machine' or some kind of **grill** to cook your meat. There are several different models. I recommend the one with the removable cooking plates. Saves a lot of clean-up. Avoid any frying.

• An **accurate bathroom scale** for your morning weighing. You need one that is accurate to within a tenth of a pound. Yes, it is important to be as **precise as possible**. Spend some money and get a good one.

Food Preparation & Presentation.

"... nothing is completely functional... unless it is beautiful to look at..."

One of my favorite art professors always used to say, "... nothing is completely functional... unless it is **beautiful** to look at!" It's really very true.

Don't overlook the importance of cooking and preparing flavorful **and** attractive foods.

Spend some time, collecting your arsenal of spices and seasonings, whose ingredients pass muster, for the **HCG + 500 phase** of your diet. Look at recipes and alluring photos of appetizing foods. A lot of the appeal of those mouth watering foods is in their 'presentation.' Your daily food consumption is limited BUT it **doesn't** have to be bland and ugly. You are on a special life changing diet, not an inmate. Have fun!

Teach yourself to prepare your meals as an appetizing and enjoyable event. Learn how to marinate and season. You will also develop a heightened sense of taste while on this diet. As you **cleanse your palate** you will really taste and enjoy your meals.

Check out the **tested** 500 Calorie **recipes** in **Section Four: 'Your Tools for Victory'**

Flow Chart of the Entire HCG Process.

"You will develop a heightened sense of taste while on this diet."

Let's look at the big picture. On the next page you will find a complete overview of the **HCG assisted weight loss cure** from **'blast off'** to **'return to earth.'**

You will journey where you have never been before and discover many new things. It is not without a cost, but if you stay the course you will return to earth a changed person and you will leave the fat behind... forever.

It's time to **prepare yourself** for the trip. The next page is **your road map to victory**. Take some time to get the overall picture, your understanding of how everything works and the order of your progression is one of the **keys to success**.

Section Three: **The 'HCG Process' FLOW CHART**

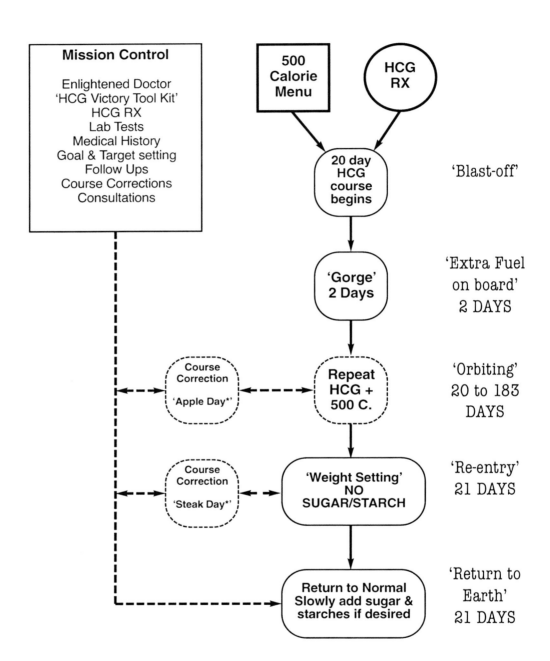

"You will journey where you have never been before and discover many new things."

"It is not without a cost, but if you stay the course you will return to earth a changed person and you will leave the fat behind... forever."

The NO Sugar No Starch Zone

That's the title of **Section Seven of the HCG Victory Guide** and it covers in detail the **'Weight Setting'** phase. It complete's your **permanent weight loss** solution.

*Details on the use of the **'apple day'** and **'steak day'** are covered at the end of **Section Seven under 'Troubleshooting,' Page 193.**

Section Four:

'Tools for YOUR Victory.'

"Refusing to be side-tracked by an all too facile interpretation of obesity, I have always held that overeating is the result of the disorder, not its cause..."

Dr. A.T.W. Simeons

Defeat OBESITY...Forever!

The HCG Assisted 500 Calorie Weight Loss Cure

Section Four: **Tools for YOUR Victory**

Equipment and Resources.

This section is a compilation of the basic tools you will need at your disposal to plan and carry out successfully the **HCG + 500 Calorie** part of Dr. Simeons plan.

"...just focus on the foods you must eat and the methodolgy used in preparing and consuming them."

You will find simplified charts of the foods that you are approved to eat within the Four Food Groups: **Protein, Vegetables, Fruits and Starches**.

No need to waste your time with the foods you can't eat, just **focus on** the foods you **must** eat and **the methodology** used in **preparing and consuming** them.

The 'Food Group Tables' are Self Explanatory.

You simply make your choices in each of the four groups remembering to rotate or alternate them and record them on the **'HCG + 500 Calorie 5 Day MEAL PLANNER'** (page 69) provided. I have included a sample already filled out so you can see how easy it is. You will note than there are 5 days on the form, this matches up with your HCG supplies of four bottles which lasts five days each, or **20 days** for **'one course'** to use the doctors terminology.

What I discovered, is you really only need to do one 5 day plan to follow, making sure that the dinner on day 5 and the lunch on day 1 are different combinations, then just simply repeat it. That worked for me. Now you have **a simple plan** to follow.

Keep Good Meal Records.

" You have a plan. The next step is to use the plan as a guide..."

You have a plan. The next step is to use the plan as a guide, but **record every meal** exactly as it happens using other copies of the blank form. So you will have a master plan and a record of how well you followed the plan. This just takes a few moments but it is **very important**. You need to know exactly what you did and when, should you at some point, need a course correction .

Here's Where the Fun Starts.

Now you need to look at the **'Vanishing Pounds and Inches'** charts on **pages 79-89**. Or as I like to call them the 'poof' charts... as in 'poof' it's gone! There is also a **space to record** other medical data, such as blood sugar or blood pressure measurements and any medication records you want to track.

"Now you need to look at the 'Vanishing Pounds and Inches' charts..."

Once again, I have included a form already filled in, based on my actual experience.

Other Tools and Tips:

Bathing & Grooming Products & Cautions.

Sugars: 'Natural' & 'Un-natural' The low down on the sweetener pitfalls.

Organic Foods: "This Doesn't Look Like Kansas Anymore... ToTo" Probably the number one buzz word in the food industry is 'organic.' Probably as a result of recent food scares the interest in 'organic' fruit, vegetables, meat, and just about everything else has gone mainstream. You will find a lot of helpful information on the subject.

'Sugar & Spice... Not Everything's Nice!' Some important do's and don'ts. Watch out for those seasonings! How to read a 'Nutrition Facts' label.

Section Four: **Bathing & Grooming CAUTIONS & Products**

The 'Midas Touch'... Not Exactly!

One of the effects of **HCG** in your system is a **hypersensitivity** to sugars, starches, oils and fats. As surprising as it sounds, when it comes to oils & fats, this extends to **even touching** or rubbing them into your skin!

Here's an excerpt from Doctor Simeons on the subject.

> "When no dietary error is elicited we turn to cosmetics. Most women find it hard to believe that fats, oils, creams and ointments applied to the skin are absorbed and interfere with weight reduction by HCG just as if they had been eaten.

> This almost **incredible sensitivity** to even such very minor increases in nutritional intake is **a peculiar feature** of the HCG method.

> For instance, we find that persons who habitually handle organic fats, such as workers in beauty parlors, masseurs, butchers, etc. never show what we consider a satisfactory loss of weight unless they can avoid fat coming into contact with their skin."

"Most women find it hard to believe that fats, oils, creams and ointments applied to the skin are absorbed and interfere..."

Wow!

So that means, during the **relatively short time** that you are ingesting the HCG hormone, you need to studiously **avoid any oils or fats either eaten or applied to your body**... and yes... the same rules apply to **men** or **anyone on HCG**.

Here's a little more **specific advice** on the 'cosmetics' question from the doctor.

> "We are particularly averse to those modern cosmetics which contain hormones, as any interference with endocrine regulations during treatment must be absolutely avoided. Many women whose skin has in the course of years become adjusted to the use of fat containing cosmetics find that their skin gets dry as soon as they stop using them. In such cases we permit the use of **plain mineral oil**, which has no nutritional value."

> "We do permit the use of **lipstick, powder** and such lotions as are entirely **free of fatty substances**. We also allow brilliantine to be used on the hair but it must not be rubbed into the scalp. Obviously sun-tan oil is prohibited."

"We are particularly averse to those modern cosmetics which contain hormones..."

Times Have Changed... Products Also.

Since Dr. Simeons era there exists an increased awareness of the residual effects of products that come in contact with our skin. In fact some entire 'cosmetic' product lines exist primarily due to the sensitivity of their clients to various ingredients.

The bottom line of all of this is **you should find it easier** to obtain products that are 'HCG friendly' and contain no fats or oils. So just like you should do when you look for spices and condiments... **read the ingredients** for the real story.

You may want to do **some special shopping** to get you by. See the short list on the next page for some general ideas and some **brand names** that are **safe**.

"...you should find it easier to obtain products that are 'HCG friendly' and contain no fats or oils."

Section Four: **Bathing & Grooming CAUTIONS & Products**

Massages.

This is another area of **potential problems** that is often not considered. Most massages use oils and lotions which **can stall your weight loss** and even result in weight gain. Doctor Simeons has some sage advice in that area.

> "I never allow any kind of massage during treatment. It is entirely unnecessary and merely disturbs a very delicate process which is going on in the tissues.

> Few indeed are the masseurs and masseuses who can resist the temptation to knead and hammer abnormal fat deposits. In the course of rapid reduction it is sometimes possible to pick up a fold of skin which has not yet had time to adjust itself, as it always does under HCG, to the changed figure.

> This fold contains its normal subcutaneous fat and may be almost an inch thick. It is one of the main objects of the HCG treatment to keep that fat there. Patients and their masseurs do not always understand this and give this fat a working-over. I have seen such patients who were as black and blue as if they had received a sound thrashing."

Want to know how he really feels? Read this.

> "How **anyone in his right mind** is able to believe that fatty tissue can be shifted mechanically or be made to vanish by squeezing is beyond my comprehension. The only effect obtained is severe bruising. The torn tissue then forms scars, and these slowly contract making the fatty tissue even harder and more unyielding."

Okay doctor, we get the picture. Time to **cancel or postpone** that massage.

"I never allow any kind of massage during treatment. It is entirely unnecessary and merely disturbs a very delicate process which is going on in the tissues."

"...exercise caution, minimize their use when on HCG, read the labels and use good old 'common sense."

Table A Bathing & Beauty Products	
Product	**Safe Brands & Suggestions**
Bathing Soaps	Dial, Ivory, Zest or Other 'Oil Free' Soaps
Cosmetics	Any 'Oil Free' Product. Use the Minimum.
Cosmetic Removers	'Oil Free' brands or 'Witch Hazel'
Deodorants	Use natural or organic chemical free products
Hair Products	Check ingredients. Excercise caution on scalp.
Lipsticks & Balms	Minimize use during HCG + 500 Calorie Phase
Lotions & Potions	For dry skin Mineral Oil used very sparingly.
Sun Tan/Sun Screen	'Oil Free' products. Mineral Oil. Minimize or eliminate.
Toothpaste	Any 'Sugar Free' brand or Baking Soda

One Final Thought.

Ladies and gentlemen, you can usually use your regular products, without a problem, as long as you exercise caution, minimize their use when on HCG, read the labels and use good old '**common sense.**' Just keep the good doctor's warnings in mind!

Section Four:

Sugars: 'Natural' & 'Un-natural'

"...each year we consume about 100 pounds of sugar per person."

One lump? or TWO?

How big is your sweet tooth? We all have one. Statistically in the USA each year we consume about **100 pounds of sugar** per person. Just to be clear, we are talking 'sugar' from sugar cane or sugar beets. About 4 ounces of the white, sparkling, sweet stuff, every day. Yes, **we eat that much** processed sugar daily!

How do we eat that much sugar you might ask? Because 'common household variety sugar' is actually not that sweet. It takes about **8 teaspoons** to sweeten one 12 ounce soft drink. It adds up fast. Sugar **enhances the taste of food**, and so not surprisingly, **an alarming number of products** contain at least some sugar.

You must **be on your guard** against 'sugar' in it's many forms and disguises. You must **keep it out** of your diet. It is a critical part of your **HCG + 500 Calorie** plan.

The **Nutrition Facts Table** found on grocery products is NOT required to list any one of these forms of sugar, if it is below 5% of the 'suggested serving size.'

"You must be on your guard against 'sugar' in it's many forms and disguises."

So as you can imagine, **companies who produce foods**, go ahead and add the 'sweetener,' since it tastes better and helps sales. This requires **manipulation** of the 'serving size' to keep the sweetener from being named on the Nutrition Facts Label.

Here are some of the aliases of sugar, **as an ingredient**, to be on the alert for:

Table B Sugar by 'Any Other Name' is Still Sugar		
Barley malt	Ethyl maltol	Malt syrup
Beet sugar	Fructose	Maltodextrin
Brown sugar	Fruit juice	Maltose
Buttered syrup	Fruit juice concentrate	Mannitol
Cane-juice crystals	galactose	Molasses
Cane sugar	Glucose	Muscovado
Caramel	Glucose solids	Panocha
Carob syrup	Golden sugar	Refiner's syrup
Corn syrup	Golden syrup	Rice Syrup
Corn syrup solids	Grape sugar	Sorbitol
Date sugar	High-fructose corn	Sorghum syrup
Demerara Sugar	syrup	Sucrose
Dextran	Honey	Sugar
Dextrose	Invert sugar	Treacle
Diatase	Lactose	Turbinado sugar
Diastatic malt	Malt	Yellow sugar

"...just go straight to the ingredients section of the product label."

Whew!

Just go straight to the **ingredients section** of the product label. There you will find **the naked truth**, albeit sometimes disguised using some of the names above. Another little trick is to use an acronym like 'HFCS' for high-fructose corn syrup.

So the bottom line is **avoid anything** that is listed as a **sugar like ingredient**!

Section Four: **Sugars: 'Natural' & 'Un-natural'**

Doctor Jekyll or Mr. Hyde?

Saccharin is an 'un-natural' sweetener that was on the scene in Dr. Simeons day, and you may have noted, was approved as a sweetener to use while on HCG.

It was discovered in 1879 and widely used until about 1972 when it was removed from the 'Generally Recognized as Safe' list in the USA, and fell into disfavor.

Even today controversy dogs many **'un-natural'** or artificial sweeteners, such as **saccharin, cyclamates, aspartame** and **sucralose**. Many of these products with catchy names like 'Equal®' and 'Splenda®,' are by volume, many times sweeter than refined sugar products.

Most of the problems evolve from **long term** and **high volume** usage.

So for the purpose of our relatively short term HCG diet plan (20 to 183 days) could be used appropriately as needed. However, many doctors and medical experts would advise you not to use these products, due to possible side effects.

All that Glitters is not Gold.

Here is what is **important** for you to successfully reach your inches and pounds goals on the **HCG assisted 500 Calorie** plan.

1) During the use of 'HCG + 500 Diet' and the 'Weight -Setting Phase' you **must not use refined sugar** products by themselves or as an ingredient. No matter how small the amount.

2) If you need some form of sweetener **use only the 'natural' sweeteners** listed below. Just stay the course, your taste buds will sharpen up and you will find that you really don't need much.

3) Use **'Natural Sweeteners'** such as Stevia, Agave Nectar or Erythritol as shown in 'Table C' below.

"...controversy dogs many 'un-natural' or artificial sweetener products..."

"...many doctors and medical experts would advise that you not use these products..."

"...your taste buds will sharpen up and you will find that you really don't need much sweetener."

Table C 'Natural' Sweetener Products		
Stevia	**Agave Nectar**	**Erythritol**
Derived from the Stevia plant.The rebiana variety is best. avaliable in liquid and granulated forms.	From the salmiana variety of the Agave plant is the best. Liquid form similar to honey with no after taste.	Sugar alcohol fermented from grapes and melons. Granulated form. Fairly new on the market.
Brand Names:	**Brand Names:**	**Brand Names:**
Steviva ® *Truvia ®* *PureVia ®*	*Madhava ®*	*Sweet Simplicity ®* *Z Sweet ®* *(also in Truvia ®)*

Section Four: **Season & Spice: Not Everything's Nice.**

All 'Facts' are NOT 'Nutritional.'

"...a few examples of the pitfalls in seasoning products..."

Here are a few examples of the **pitfalls** in seasoning products, taken right from the 'Nutrition Label' on a few I found in my cupboard. Using seasoning with sugar when using HCG can **sabotage** your **results**. It pays to **read** the labels **very carefully**.

Not trying to pick on just these companies, the practices, of what I would call **'label manipulation,'** are very widespread. They follow the 'letter' of the law but not the 'spirit' of the law. You and I, are the worse for it.

Case One:

Durkee Grill Creations

Citrus Grill Seasoning

"...the practices, of what I would call 'label manipulation,' are very widespread."

Ooops! Hidden Sugars & Starches

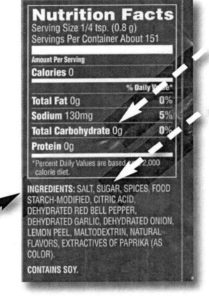

Hmmm... Nothing Here?

High Sugar Content!

Ingredients are listed in descending order, with the most being first.

Sugar is listed as the number 2 ingredient and Starch is number 3.

Contains both Sugar and Starch. Avoid this type of seasoning!

Case Two:

McCormick Garlic Salt with Parsley

No MSG

"They follow the 'letter' of the law but not the 'spirit' of the law. You and I are the worse for it."

Note: Hidden Sugars & Starches

Modified Corn Starch is listed as the number 2 ingredient, Garlic is 3, Sugar is number 4.

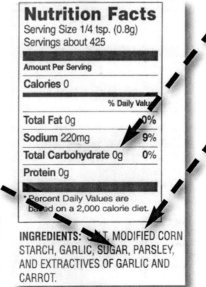

Don't see... Anything Listed Here?

High Starch Content!

Ingredients are listed in descending order, with the most being first.

Contains both Sugar and Starch. Avoid this type of seasoning!

Section Four: **Season & Spice: Not Everything's Nice.**

Always Check the INGREDIENTS.

"The information in the 'Nutrition Facts Label' can be misleading."

The information on the '**Nutrition Facts**' label, can be **misleading**. For instance, if the size of the '**suggested serving**' is manipulated so that the sugar content is less than 5%, then it is not required to be listed. However, that sugar content, will be **a problem** while you are participating in the **HCG protocol**.

Below is a label from an '**HCG safe**' seasoning product. Note the absence of sugar or starch of any kind in the **ingredients** listing. Below is a short list of some brands of safe seasonings. You can easily locate what you need, just read labels carefully.

Case Three:

Simply Organic Grilling Seasons Steak Seasoning

USDA Organic

"Note the absence of sugar or starch of any kind in the ingredients listing."

Aha!
At last we have a seasoning that is **COMPLETELY SAFE** for you to use during your **HCG + 500 Calorie** and **NO sugar NO starch** phases.

INGREDIENTS: SEA SALT, ORGANIC ONION, ORGANIC GARLIC, ORGANIC BLACK PEPPER, ORGANIC THYME, ORGANIC TARRAGON, ORGANIC BAY LEAF.

Nutrition Facts
Serv. Size: 1/4 tsp (0.8g),
Servings: 125 Amount Per Serving: **Calories** 0, **Total Fat** 0g (0% DV), **Sodium** 90mg (4% DV), **Total Carbohydrate** 0g (0% DV), **Protein** 0g, Not a significant source of calories from fat, saturated fat, trans fat, cholesterol, dietary fiber, sugars, vitamin A, vitamin C, calcium, and iron. Percent Daily Values (DV) are based on a 2,000 calorie diet.

Note: NO Hidden Sugars NO Hidden Starches

USDA Organic means that 95% of the ingredients used in the product are certified to be organic

---

Table D   A Short List of 'HCG Safe' Seasonings

Product	Safe Brands & Suggestions
All Natural Seasonings	Kelly's Original, Onion or Garlic
Dill Weed	Spice Islands 100% Organic
Garlic Salt	5th Season, Simply Organic
Ground Celery Salt	Tradewinds
Onion Salt	McCormick
Poultry Seasoning	Frontier Natural Products
Steak Seasoning	Simply Organic

"... you can easily locate what you need."

Your Shopping List.

You can find these products just about anywhere, although the 'health foods' store will have the biggest variety. Once you try these seasonings you just may like them.

Going, Going, Gone Organic.

Young Dorothy and her little doggie, found themselves whisked away to the land of OZ, where among other things, she learned that all questions would be answered if she just "...followed the **'yellow brick road.'** We all know how that turned out.

The 'Wizard' turned out to be a phony and a fake and the Emerald City... well, it just wasn't what it appeared to be. In the end it was all just one big dream... or was it?

We have all been following our own 'yellow brick road,' trusting the bureaucrats and the **big food companies** to take care of everything. Now much of our food supply is 'phoney' and 'fake' and isn't good for us. It **looks good** but is **mainly a facade**.

"Now much of our food supply is 'phoney' and 'fake' and isn't good for us.

There is No Place Like Home.

Organic growers, farmers and food producers are attempting to get us back home on the farm, away from the nearly **600 pesticides** used in agriculture production. Synthetic chemicals are in everything we eat. More safety concerns appear daily.

Organic farmers believe that the strongest plants and healthiest livestock thrive without the added chemicals. Thus the 'organic' industry avoids these practices.

Just as learning how to eat healthy is important to your body's health, so to, is what kind of food you eat. Garbage in... garbage out. **Eat a chemical... be a chemical.**

"...learning how to eat healthy is important to your body's health."

Somewhere Over the Rainbow.

Have you ever tasted a vine ripened tomato picked at it's peak after being allowed to ripen in it's own time? How about a tree ripened apple or peach? The same concept is true of farm animals who are allowed to grow at their own natural pace without artificial stimulants or hormones. That's what 'organic food' is all about.

As it turns out, there is **a direct connection** between **flavor** and **nutrition**.

Nutrient rich soil, clean water, good feed, healthy pastures. Not surprising is it?

Courage, Brains, and a Heart.

In my opinion you should choose **organic** products for the foods you eat day in and day out. Patronize **your local organic farm** producers. Check out **Section Six & Seven** of your 'tool kit' for **web sites** to locate organically produced products.

"...you should choose organic products for the foods you eat day in and day out."

If you have any doubts about the **increased nutritional values** in organic foods, check out the facts and figures via the previously referenced web sites.**(p.168-69)**

Having all of the **chemical influences** absorbed into our body from **non-organic** foods no doubt **contributes to** our obesity problem by **altering** our **sensitive natural weight management** system.

If you use your **brain**, you know, **it is smart** to eat **organic**.

In your **heart**, you know it's the right thing to do. Especially for the foods you eat most often. **Be courageous** and do the right thing. Don't fear the 'flying monkeys.'

There really is '...no place like home!'

HCG + 500 CALORIES

FOUR FOOD GROUPS

Section Four: Food Group 1: Proteins for Victory

The first group you need to become familiar with is 'proteins.' Dr. Simeons '500 calorie course' as he refers to it, is 40% protein driven. Understanding and using them properly is a critical element in assuring your success with the HCG + 500 Calorie protocol. Think of it as your formula for victory. Win with proper protein management... lose control without it!

Nothing that the good doctor recommends is by accident. He discovered over 40 years the proper balance and the food group usage. The charts that follow are streamlined so that you can put together your meal plans as easily as possible.

You and I are no different than any other person who has succeeded with this amazing HCG assisted protocol. Protein in the right amount and rotation is key. Do it right and you will most assuredly win. Don't worry about what you 'can't' eat, focus instead on what you MUST eat for victory.

Emphasis is on the foods you CAN eat in your 500 Calorie HCG assisted phase, with a few clarifying exceptions.

NOTE: Remember ALL weight references for MEATS in the protein group are in RAW ounces. Dr. Simeon references 100 grams in his manuscript which is equal to 3.75 ounces. You must learn how to weigh your meat, a postal scale works fine.

Description	HCG 500	NS/NS		Life	Serving Size	Calories	Protein	Fat	SatFat	Notes:
Ground Beef	NO	Y	Y	Y	3.75 oz	300	25	0	15	6
Filet Mignon	Caution	Y	Y	Y	3.75 oz	240	25	0	9	3
Flank Steak	YES	Y	Y	Y	3.75 oz	210	24	0	6	3
Rib Steak	YES	Y	Y	Y	3.75 oz	210	24	0	7	3
Rib Pot Roast	YES	Y	Y	Y	3.75 oz	175	15	0	7	3
Roast, lean	Caution	Y	Y	Y	3.75 oz	240	30	0	6	2
Round Steak	YES	Y	Y	Y	3.75 oz	185	25	0	3	1
Sirloin Steak	YES	Y	Y	Y	3.75 oz	300	22	0	16	6

This list of beef is easily obtained at your supermarket or co-op. Many meat departments feature 'thin cut' or 'petite' steaks which will be about 3.75 ounces when trimmed. Don't forget...we TRIM ALL VISIBLE FAT before weighing and cooking.

Description	HCG 500	NS/NS		Life	Serving Size	Calories	Protein	Fat	SatFat	Notes:
LAMB	NO	Y	Y	Y	3.75 oz	170	22	8	4	1

Description	HCG 500	NS/NS		Life	Serving Size	Calories	Protein	Fat	SatFat	Notes:
PORK	NO	Y	Y	Y	3.75 oz	150	22	6	3	1

Lamb and Pork are NOT APPROVED for the 500 Calorie HCG assisted phase. Very important to trust the old doctor on this and avoid these two protein sources at this point. Later you will be able to add them back in after you have reached your pounds and inches goals.

Description	HCG 500	NS/NS		Life	Serving Size	Calories	Protein	Fat	SatFat	Notes:
Chicken Eggs	YES	Y	Y	Y	One Large	75	6	0	5	2
Chicken Breast	YES	Y	Y	Y	3.75 oz	85	14	0	0	0

These are the only poultry protein sources approved to begin your diet. The chicken breast is skinless either fresh or frozen. ALL VISIBLE FAT is trimmed of course, and weighed RAW. Cooking method is grilled. Watch out for cooking sprays and avoid frying or oils of any kind. Seasonings are OK, but revisit pages 52-53 for tips, ideas and cautions.

Section Four: Food Group 1: Proteins for Victory

Description	HCG 500	NS/NS	Life	Serving Size	Calories	Protein	Fat	SatFat	Notes:
Ground Veal (8%)	YES	Y	Y Y	3.75 oz	190	26	6	3	
Veal Round Steak	YES	Y	Y Y	3.75 oz	175	25	3	1	
Lean Veal Roast	YES	Y	Y Y	3.75 oz	130	15	7	3	
Veal S. Ribs, lean	YES	Y	Y Y	3.75 oz	65	7	5	2	

These are the only veal choices at the beginning, ALL VISIBLE FAT is trimmed of course, and weighed RAW. Cooking method is grilled, roasted or broiled. Watch out for cooking sprays and avoid frying or oils of any kind. Seasoning is OK but check out pages 52-53 for tips and ideas.

Description	HCG 500	NS/NS	Life	Serving Size	Calories	Protein	Fat	SatFat	Notes:
Fish, (Low Fat) Approved 'fish' varieties that are Low Fat & Low Calorie are: Bass, Cod, Flounder, Grouper, Haddock, Ling, Monkfish, Northern Pike, Ocean Perch, Orange Roughy, Pike, Pollock, Rockfish, Rainbow Smelt, Snapper, Sole, Tilapia, Whiting & Wolffish.	YES	Y	Y Y	3.75 oz	80-110	10-30	1-3	0	Caution
Shellfish: Crab	YES	Y	Y Y	3.75 oz	80-120	18	0-2	0-1	
Shellfish: Crayfish	YES	Y	Y Y	3.75 oz	75	15	1	0	
Shellfish: Lobster	YES	Y	Y Y	3.75 oz	100	20	1	0	
Scallops	Caution	Y	Y Y	3.75 oz	100	18	1	0	
Shrimp	YES	Y	Y Y	3.75 oz	125	25	2	0	

SOME NECESSARY PRECAUTIONS: Approach the seafood category cautiously, as some people find that for them personally, seafood drastically slows or prevents their weight loss rate when on the 500 Calorie HCG assisted portion of the diet. Many people are also allergic to shellfish as a category.

There are many other types of fish and seafood out there, but you must confine yourself to CAUTIOUSLY using those listed here. Remember we are focusing on what you CAN eat and what is EASILY AVAILABLE, not what you CANNOT, eat or find.

CHECK THE LABELS on your favorite fish sauce carefully for ANY kind of sugar additives! All kinds of seasonings are OK, but read the ingredients carefully. Once again, for guidelines check out pages 52-53 for tips and ideas.

When checking labels, LOOK FIRST at all listed INGREDIENTS. Product creators do not have to list 'sugar' as an ingredient on their 'Nutrition Facts' label, if it is less than 5% of the 'suggested serving.' In fact they can claim it is 'sugar free.' Watch out for this trap as they will often manipulate the serving size to make their product appear to be 'sugar free.'

All INGREDIENTS must be listed however, and if there is any form of SUGAR or CORN SYRUP in the product, the 'Ingredients:" is where you will discover it. Remember 'sugars' and 'oils,' in any form and in any amount, in what you are eating in the 500 Calorie HCG assisted diet phase, WILL NEGATIVELY AFFECT YOUR PROGRESS, or stop it all together!

COOKING METHODS are grilling, steaming, barbecueing or broiling. Watch out for cooking sprays and avoid frying or oils of any kind. You should be keeping 'eating records' and they will be very helpful should you lose your way.

Section Four: Food Group 2: Vegetables for Victory

Vegetables are the second food group that we need for our daily menu choices. Vegetables are the main source for a wide variety of vitamins and minerals. I have streamlined your choices, once again focusing on those varieties approved and painstakingly tested through trial and error, by Dr. Simeons.

You don't need an endless list of forbidden veggies. Here is the list you CAN choose from to fit your palate and still stay on track for your weight loss victory dance. You are planning one aren't you? Maybe you have been dreaming about losing weight for years and you just can't imagine the joy you will be feeling when you finally make it...well...victory is now within your grasp. Check out the list of vegetables below and pick your favorites. Note: A slight change on the table below, 'Carbs' and 'Fiber' replace the 'Fat' and 'Sat Fat' columns since that is more appropriate when looking at veggies.

Description	HCG 500	NS/NS Life	Serving Size	Calories	Protein	Sugar	Carbs	Fiber
Asparagus	YES	Y Y Y	4 oz.	25	3	1	5	2
Cabbage	YES	Y Y Y	1 cup	27	2	3	6	2
Celery	YES	Y Y Y	1 cup	17	1	1	4	2
Cucumbers	YES	Y Y Y	1 cup	16	1	2	3	1
Lettuces, all	YES	Y Y Y	1 cup	21	2	2	4	2
Onion, small	YES	Y Y Y	one	29	1	3	7	1
Red Radishes	YES	Y Y Y	1/2 cup	15	1	1	1	1
Spinach, cooked	YES	Y Y Y	1 cup	41	5	1	7	4
Spinach, raw	YES	Y Y Y	1 cup	11	1	0	3	1
Tomatoes, cherry	YES	Y Y Y	1 cup	27	1	4	6	2
Tomatoes, medium	YES	Y Y Y	one	35	1	5	7	1

When choosing vegetables for your menu, BE SURE TO ROTATE THEM so that you don't use the same one twice in a row.

Also another precaution is in order...TOMATOES are another potential weight-loss stopper, so approach their use cautiously. Be sure to track what you are eating and weigh in every morning at the same time, that way you will spot any approved foods that are not working for you and correct course. After your first 20 days you can experiment with a little mixing.

Food Group 3: Fruits for Victory

Description	HCG 500	NS/NS Life	Serving Size	Calories	Protein	Sugar	Carbs	Fiber
Apples, large	YES	Y Y Y	one	75	0	14	19	3
Grapefruit, all	YES	Y Y Y	1/2 medium	60	1	10	16	5
Lemons, medium	YES	Y Y Y	one daily	15	0	1	5	1
Oranges, medium	YES	Y Y Y	one	70	1	12	16	3
Tangerines, med	YES	Y Y Y	one	50	1	8	13	3

Fruits are the third part of the formula. ORGANIC fruits are always recommended. Your choice of Apples, and in this group, they are the 'workhorse' fruit, . They can be baked or fried, eaten fresh or go wonderfully in a salad. You will note that all of the other fruits the good doctor recommends are citrus based. Does that make you wonder where all of the 'grapefruit' diets got the idea? Apparently the approved 'citrus' varieties help to burn the fat in the right way. BERRIES of all kinds are NOT included at this point, probably due to their higher sugar content.

Be aware that ORANGES can be a LOSS STOPPER for some people. This seems to vary from one person to another.

Section Four: Food Group 4: 'Starches' for Victory

BREADS	HCG 500	NS/NS	Life	Serving Size	Calories	Protein	Sugar	Carbs	Fiber
Melba Toast	YES	Y Y	Y	one round	20	0	0	0	0
Breadstick		Y Y	Y	one	20	0	0	0	0

If you must have it these are the allowed 'bread' products for the 500 Calorie HCG assisted diet. The doctor recommends you eat very small amounts of this type of starch.

The breadsticks that are recommended are called 'grissini' and I did find them difficult to locate.

Approved BEVERAGES

BEVERAGES	HCG 500	NS/NS	Life	Serving Size	Calories	Protein	Sugar	Carbs	Fiber
Coffee	YES	Y Y	Y	8 oz.	10	0	0	0	0
Tea	YES	Y Y	Y	8 oz.	2	0	0	0	0
Mineral Water	YES	Y Y	Y	8 oz.	0	0	0	0	0
Pure Water	YES	Y Y	Y	8 oz.	0	0	0	0	0

The DAILY INTAKE of plenty of fluids is important. Your goal should be to drink about 68 OUNCES a day. That sounds like a lot but, when you consider that the average glass or coffee cup holds 8 to 10 ounces, it is easy to accomplish. Most bottled water is 12 or 16 ounces. A large cup of (black all the way to the top) espresso is 20 ounces.

You may drink your beverages, whenever you want and in any quantity, throughout the day. Poor fluid intake can stall you.

NO CREAM OR SUGAR or any other sugar based additives. Sugar substitutes such as 'Stevia' and 'Guava Nectar' are allowed and really taste fine. Check 'Sugars: 'Natural and Un-natural' on pages 50-51 for ideas, suggestions and cautions.

'Wild Cards'

MISCELLANEOUS	HCG 500	NS/NS	Life	Serving Size	Calories	Protein	Sugar	Carbs	Fat/Sat
Cottage Cheese	YES	Y Y	Y	1/4 cup	58	7	0	2	3/2
Milk	YES	Y Y	Y	1 Tbsp	2	0	0	0	0
Soup, Broth	YES	Y Y	Y	1 cup	0	0	0	0	0
Vinegars	YES	Y Y	Y	8 oz.	3	0	0	1	0

These are some foods that don't fit neatly into one category. Cottage cheese has some protein value. Milk is allowed but in very small amounts. Beef or chicken broth, as a soup or a soup base, are allowed. Organic natural vinegar is very useful as a salad dressing.

Check out all of the great, safe ideas for use with the '500 Calorie + HCG recipes' on pages 91-98.

OH NO!

WEIGHTS
&
MEASURES

WEIGHTS & MEASURES

ISBN 978-0-9800641-7-9

Section Four: **Oh No! Weights & Measures**

Now Entering the Olympic Stadium.

If you are preparing for the next Olympics you need to be **very** lean with maybe two to three percent body fat. That would make you in the top, teeny...tiny per cent, of people in the entire world. Think of Olympic swimmer and gold medal winner **Michael Phelps**. Good luck if you aspire to that standard!

For the rest of us, that would be 99.9% of us who **aspire to be normal**, we need to find our normal range. This is where it gets sticky. What is normal?

Who's On First?

When was the last time you felt like your weight and overall health was great and you felt great? That should be a clue to what your normal 'weight range' should be.

Why do I use the term **'range?'** Well here is a diagram that illustrates an important personal weight concept. You guessed it... **we are all different**.

"...we need to find our normal range."

"When was the last time you felt like your weight and overall health was great... that should be a clue."

Table E   Example Male 6' 0" Weight Range

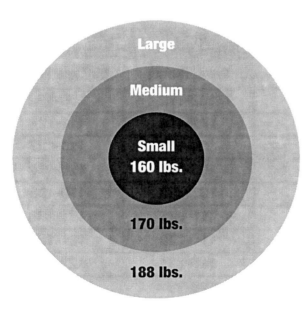

Large

Medium

Small
160 lbs.

170 lbs.

188 lbs.

Believe it or Dare.

Here's a summary of a number of 'experts' opinions on what I should weigh...

...OK, you can stop laughing anytime.

Most of the 'weight tables' I have studied are developed by 'insurance' companies or their affiliates. Let's see now, their goal is not to help you find the right weight, their goal is to develop a table with the lowest possible 'mortality rate,' because they use that to justify raising their rates. Hmmm.

Age, fitness level, muscle mass and lifestyle are hardly reflected in these hypothetical calculations... sheesh!

Remember these are AVERAGES.

I Was Framed!

What is your frame size? If you don't know if you are small, medium or large here's **a simple way** to determine that. If you are right handed use that hand to measure your left wrist, or do the reverse if you are a southpaw.

Section Four: **Oh No! Weights & Measures**

Take your thumb and middle finger (yes that naughty finger) and try to reach around your wrist at the **narrow point** right before your hand, right after that boney bump.

Unless you have more than two arms there are just three possibilities:

Middle finger **overlaps** your thumb:	SMALL FRAME
Middle finger **barely touches** your thumb:	MEDIUM FRAME
A **gap** between middle finger and thumb:	LARGE FRAME

"It's not rocket science but it does give you a general idea."

Well what did you expect? It's not rocket science but it does give you an idea.

Tongue in Cheek 'Please Weigh Me' Tables.

Here are a couple of composite charts to use as a guide. If you stop and think about it, you know what your normal should be. Don't let the charts knock you for a loop. Personally I couldn't stop laughing. I haven't weighed 170 lbs. since I was in high school and I was all skin and bones. Who are these people? Oh well, never mind.

So with that thought in mind and tongue in cheek, I am listing a **range** of weights for men and women. Probably most of you are going to be shooting for the high end of the range and that's OK. Here we go, **ladies first**.

"Probably most people are going to be on the high end and that's OK."

"Consultation with your physician is the best way to get a realistic goal."

Table F Weight Range for WOMEN by Frame Size			
Height	**Small Frame**	**Medium Frame**	**Large Frame**
4'10"	102-112	109-122	131-136
4'11"	103-114	111-124	134-139
5'0"	104-116	113-127	137-142
5'1"	106-119	115-130	140-145
5'2"	108-122	118-133	143-148
5'3"	111-125	121-136	147-152
5'4"	114-128	124-139	151-156
5'5"	117-131	127-142	155-160
5'6"	120-134	130-145	159-164
5'7"	123-137	133-147	163-168
5'8"	126-140	136-150	167-172
5'9"	129-143	139-153	170-175
5'10"	132-146	142-156	173-178
5'11"	135-149	145-159	176-181
6'0"	138-152	148-162	179-184

Please note that these are compiled estimates for setting general goals.
Consultation with your physician is the best way to set your own personal and realistic goal.

Section Four: **Oh No! Weights & Measures**

OK Guys... Here's the Good News.

Remember these are guidelines. Averages compiled from statistics. For the record, **Michael Phelps** is 6' 4" and weighs 195, and he has a drawer full of gold medals. Think about that. He is all muscle and bone and he is just in the middle of the 188-208 group. Relax. Use this as a guide to help you succeed, not as an iron clad rule.

"Remember these are guidelines."

"Use this as a guide to help you succeed, not as an iron-clad rule."

Table G Weight Range for MEN by Frame Size			
Height	**Small Frame**	**Medium Frame**	**Large Frame**
5' 2"	128-135	131-142	138-151
5' 3"	130-137	133-144	140-154
5' 4"	132-139	135-146	142-157
5' 5"	134-141	137-149	144-161
5' 6"	136-143	139-152	143-165
5' 7"	138-145	142-155	149-169
5' 8"	140-149	145-158	152-173
5' 9"	142-152	148-160	155-177
5' 10"	144-155	151-164	158-181
5' 11"	146-158	154-167	161-185
6' 0"	149-161	157-170	164-189
6' 1"	152-165	160-175	168-193
6' 2"	155-169	164-179	172-198
6' 3"	158-173	167-183	176-203
6' 4"	162-177	171-188	181-208

Please note that these are compiled estimates for setting general goals.
Consultation with your physician is the best way to set your own personal and realistic goal.

Are You Ready for the Test?

Forget about it. Nobody is judging you. I am just trying to help you find some goals that are realistic for you. Many other **medical conditions**, **measurements** and features are 'normal' for you. Work with **your doctor**, review **your medical history**, examine your life, and critique your obesity problem. When did it first appear? How did you feel before and what did you weigh? These are all clues to help determine your 'weight and inches' goals. The **HCG + 500 Calorie** diet is kind of self limiting, your weight will reach a point where the **'warehouse'** is just about empty. You will know you are there. Your **weight and size** will stabilize, you will be ready to stop.

First Your Pounds... Then Your Inches.

As the **pounds** melt away the **inches will follow** along, since the fat you are burning is probably the main contributor to the size of things. Just be patient.

ISBN 978-0-9800641-7-9

CHARTS

FOR MENU PLANNING & RECORD KEEPING

MENU PLANS & RECORDS

Section Four: **MENU Planning & Charts for RECORD Keeping**

Setting Your Course.

We have covered a lot of material to this point to help you win the battle. Now it's **time to plan** your meals around the 500 Calorie plan and set your course and stay on it. Below is a partial copy of the '**HCG + 500 Calorie 5 Day Meal Planner.**'

"...it's time to plan your meals around the 500 Calorie plan"

"I found the best approach was to pre-plan the meals using the Food Tables found at the beginning of this chapter."

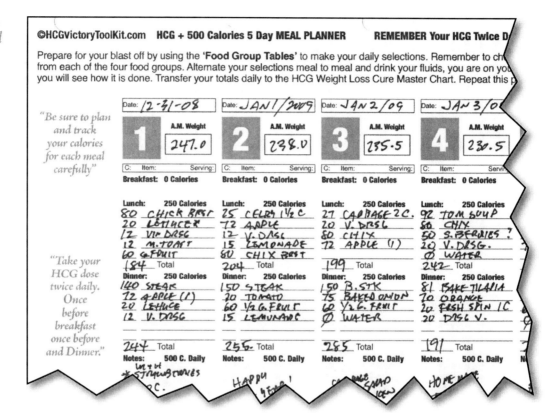

"Be sure to plan and track your calories for each meal carefully"

"Take your HCG dose twice daily. Once before breakfast once before and Dinner."

"Once you have a few 5 day plans that you have tested and you like you can just repeat them as often as needed..."

Simplicity is the keyword in this 'Tool Kit.'

I found the best approach was to **pre-plan** the meals using the **Food Tables** found at the beginning of this chapter. With the use of these tables, carefully put together your daily meals. It may help to **review** the pages on '**The 500 Calorie + HCG Diet'** found at the beginning of '**Section Three: Your Plan for Victory.'** (pages 40-44)

You will find **4 copies**, of the one sided form above, in the pages ahead. Each one covers **5 days**, which matches up with your HCG supply, you are mixing in 5 day amounts. Before you use all of the forms go ahead and **make some blank copies**, for **your personal use**, as many as you need. See how I did it, above.

Checking out the **recipes, tips and techniques** at the end of this section, for meal ideas' may help as you get started. A time saver is to just **repeat** your selections being careful to **alternate and rotate** your protein, fruit, and vegetable choices.

Once you have a few **5 day plans** that you have tested and like, you can just **repeat** them, as often as needed, with this **caution.** Be sure that the 'Day 5' and 'Day 1' choices are **not** the same. For example, the last protein for Day 5 and the first one for 'Day 1' aren't in the same food group. **Keep the rotation going.**

Section Four: **MENU Planning & Charts for RECORD Keeping**

Finding Your Way Back.

Going on a journey is no fun if you don't know where you have been, or how to get back on course, if you get lost. You need to **keep track** of where you have gone to **find your way back**. This is fundamental. Ship captains and explorers keep a log.

Your journey into 'HCG-land' is no different. You are going into, what is for you, uncharted territory. I have gone before you and have spent a lot of time simplifying and distilling, Dr. Simeons HCG protocol, down to the bare essence.

One of the **keys to victory** is to log everything you do and record your successes and failures faithfully so that if you get lost **you and your doctor** can get you back on the right track. This system **does require your focus** for maximum success.

"You need to keep track of where you have gone to find your way back..."

"One of the keys to victory is to log everything you do and record your successes and failures faithfully..."

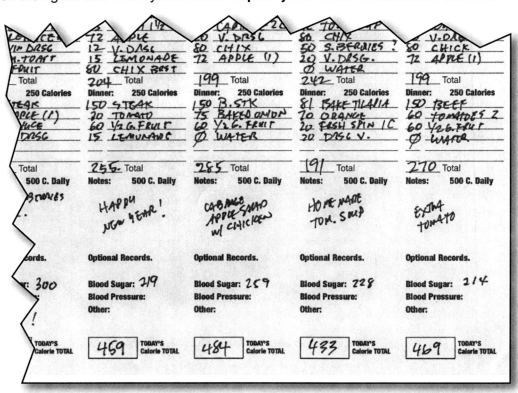

Your Brain is Required.

Boy is that true... in more ways than one. Please take the time to **learn how** to fill out these forms. Shown above is a partial, bottom section, of the meal planner.

You will note on the meal planner that you should **record the date**, record your morning **weight** daily. There is also a spot for daily **'notes'** and **'optional'** health readings. Be sure to **do all of this daily**. Weigh in at the same time in your birthday suit. Do any other testing or measuring at that time. Then **write it down**.

"Be sure to do all of this daily."

'Poof' it's Gone.

The **fun starts** when you begin to transfer your lost 'pounds and inches' and other measurements to the **'Vanishing Pounds & Inches'** chart found in the following pages, then you will recap on to your **'Poof it's Gone'** Recap form. Wow.

©HCGVictoryToolKit.com   HCG + 500 Calories 5 Day MEAL PLANNER   REMEMBER Your HCG Twice Daily!   Daily CALORIE TARGET: 500

Prepare for your blast off by using the **'Food Group Tables'** to make your daily selections. Remember to choose one item for each of your 2 daily meals from each of the four food groups. Alternate your selections meal to meal and drink your fluids, you are on your way. Check out the example included and you will see how it is done. Transfer your totals daily to the HCG Weight Loss Cure Master Chart. Repeat this plan 3 more times for a 20 day course.

"Be sure to plan and track your calories for each meal carefully"

"Take your HCG dose twice daily. Once before breakfast once before and Dinner".

"Weigh yourself in your 'birthday suit' ONE time every morning at the same time".

"Use the 'Food Tables' to plan your caloric intake in the four food groups"

"Take your HCG dose twice daily. Once before breakfast once before and Dinner".

"Use the 'Optionl Records' section if you need to track other health issues"

	1	2	3	4	5
Date:					
A.M. Weight					
C: Item: / Serving:					
Breakfast:	0 Calories	0 Calories	0 Calories	0 Calories	0 Calories
Lunch:	250 Calories	250 Calories	250 Calories	250 Calories	250 Calories
Total					
Dinner:	250 Calories	250 Calories	250 Calories	250 Calories	250 Calories
Total					
Notes:	500 C. Daily	500 C. Daily	500 C. Daily	500 C. Daily	500 C. Daily

Optional Records.	Optional Records.	Optional Records.	Optional Records.	Optional Records.
Blood Sugar:	Blood Sugar:	Blood Sugar:	Blood Sugar:	Blood Sugar:
Blood Pressure:	Blood Pressure:	Blood Pressure:	Blood Pressure:	Blood Pressure:
Other:	Other:	Other:	Other:	Other:
TODAY'S Calorie TOTAL	TODAY'S Calorie TOTAL	TODAY'S Calorie TOTAL	TODAY'S Calorie TOTAL	TODAY'S Calorie TOTAL

©HCGVictoryToolKit.com   HCG + 500 Calories 5 Day MEAL PLANNER   REMEMBER Your HCG Twice Daily!   Daily CALORIE TARGET: 500

Prepare for your blast off by using the 'Food Group Tables' to make your daily selections. Remember to choose one item for each of your 2 daily meals from each of the four food groups. Alternate your selections meal to meal and drink your fluids, you are on your way. Check out the example included and you will see how it is done. Transfer your totals daily to the HCG Weight Loss Cure Master Chart. Repeat this plan 3 more times for a 20 day course.

"Be sure to plan and track your calories for each meal carefully"

"Use the 'Food Tables' to plan your calorie intake in the four food groups"

1 — Date: _____ — A.M. Weight _____

2 — Date: _____ — A.M. Weight _____

3 — Date: _____ — A.M. Weight _____

4 — Date: _____ — A.M. Weight _____

5 — Date: _____ — A.M. Weight _____

C: _____ Item: _____ Serving: _____ (each day)

Breakfast: 0 Calories

Lunch: 250 Calories

Total

Dinner: 250 Calories

Total

Notes: 500 C. Daily

"Take your HCG dose twice daily. Once before breakfast once before and Dinner."

Optional Records.

Blood Sugar:

Blood Pressure:

Other:

TODAY'S Calorie TOTAL

"Weigh yourself in your 'birthday suit' ONE time every morning at the same time."

"Use the 'Optional Records' section if you need to track other health issues"

©HCGVictoryToolKit.com   **HCG + 500 Calories 5 Day MEAL PLANNER**   **REMEMBER Your HCG Twice Daily!**   **Daily CALORIE TARGET: 500**

Prepare for your blast off by using the **'Food Group Tables'** to make your daily selections. Remember to choose one item for each of your 2 daily meals from each of the four food groups. Alternate your selections meal to meal and drink your fluids, you are on your way. Check out the example included and you will see how it is done. Transfer your totals daily to the HCG Weight Loss Cure Master Chart. Repeat this plan 3 more times for a 20 day course.

"Be sure to plan and track your calories for each meal carefully"

"Take your HCG dose twice daily. Once before breakfast once before and Dinner".

"Weigh yourself in your 'birthday suit' ONE time every morning at the same time"

"Use the 'Food Tables' to plan your calorie in-take in the four food groups"

"Take your HCG dose twice daily. Once before breakfast once before and Dinner."

"Use the 'Optional Records' section if you need to track other health issues"

Day 1

Date: _____

A.M. Weight: _____

C: _____ Item: _____ Serving: _____

Breakfast: 0 Calories

Lunch: _____ 250 Calories

_____
_____
_____
Total

Dinner: _____ 250 Calories

_____
_____
_____
Total

Notes: _____ **500 C. Daily**

Day 2

Date: _____

A.M. Weight: _____

C: _____ Item: _____ Serving: _____

Breakfast: 0 Calories

Lunch: _____ 250 Calories

_____
_____
_____
Total

Dinner: _____ 250 Calories

_____
_____
_____
Total

Notes: _____ **500 C. Daily**

Day 3

Date: _____

A.M. Weight: _____

C: _____ Item: _____ Serving: _____

Breakfast: 0 Calories

Lunch: _____ 250 Calories

_____
_____
_____
Total

Dinner: _____ 250 Calories

_____
_____
_____
Total

Notes: _____ **500 C. Daily**

Day 4

Date: _____

A.M. Weight: _____

C: _____ Item: _____ Serving: _____

Breakfast: 0 Calories

Lunch: _____ 250 Calories

_____
_____
_____
Total

Dinner: _____ 250 Calories

_____
_____
_____
Total

Notes: _____ **500 C. Daily**

Day 5

Date: _____

A.M. Weight: _____

C: _____ Item: _____ Serving: _____

Breakfast: 0 Calories

Lunch: _____ 250 Calories

_____
_____
_____
Total

Dinner: _____ 250 Calories

_____
_____
_____
Total

Notes: _____ **500 C. Daily**

Optional Records (Day 1)
Optional Records.
Blood Sugar: _____
Blood Pressure: _____
Other: _____
TODAY'S Calorie TOTAL _____

Optional Records (Day 2)
Optional Records.
Blood Sugar: _____
Blood Pressure: _____
Other: _____
TODAY'S Calorie TOTAL _____

Optional Records (Day 3)
Optional Records.
Blood Sugar: _____
Blood Pressure: _____
Other: _____
TODAY'S Calorie TOTAL _____

Optional Records (Day 4)
Optional Records.
Blood Sugar: _____
Blood Pressure: _____
Other: _____
TODAY'S Calorie TOTAL _____

Optional Records (Day 5)
Optional Records.
Blood Sugar: _____
Blood Pressure: _____
Other: _____
TODAY'S Calorie TOTAL _____

HCG + 500 Calories 5 Day MEAL PLANNER   REMEMBER Your HCG Twice Daily!   Daily CALORIE TARGET: 500

Prepare for your blast off by using the 'Food Group Tables' to make your daily selections. Remember to choose one item for each of your 2 daily meals from each of the four food groups. Alternate your selections meal to meal and drink your fluids, you are on your way. Check out the example included and you will see how it is done. Transfer your totals daily to the HCG Weight Loss Cure Master Chart. Repeat this plan 3 more times for a 20 day course.

"Be sure to plan and track your calories for each meal carefully"

"Use the 'Food Tables' to make your calorie intake in the four food groups"

1 — Date: _____ A.M. Weight ____

C: _____ Item: _____ Serving: _____
Breakfast: 0 Calories

Lunch: _____
_____
_____
_____
_____
_____ Total **250 Calories**

Dinner: _____
_____
_____
_____
_____
_____ Total **250 Calories**

Notes: _____ **500 C. Daily**

2 — Date: _____ A.M. Weight ____

C: _____ Item: _____ Serving: _____
Breakfast: 0 Calories

Lunch: **250 Calories**

Dinner: _____ Total **250 Calories**

_____ Total **500 C. Daily**

3 — Date: _____ A.M. Weight ____

C: _____ Item: _____ Serving: _____
Breakfast: 0 Calories

Lunch: **250 Calories**

Dinner: _____ Total **250 Calories**

Notes: _____ Total **500 C. Daily**

4 — Date: _____ A.M. Weight ____

C: _____ Item: _____ Serving: _____
Breakfast: 0 Calories

Lunch: **250 Calories**

Dinner: _____ Total **250 Calories**

Notes: _____ Total **500 C. Daily**

5 — Date: _____ A.M. Weight ____

C: _____ Item: _____ Serving: _____
Breakfast: 0 Calories

Lunch: **250 Calories**

Dinner: Total **250 Calories**

Notes: _____ Total **500 C. Daily**

"Take your HCG dose twice daily. Once before breakfast once before and Dinner."

"Take your HCG dose twice daily. Once before breakfast once before and Dinner."

Optional Records.
Blood Sugar:
Blood Pressure:
Other:
TODAY'S Calorie TOTAL ____

Optional Records.
Blood Sugar:
Blood Pressure:
Other:
TODAY'S Calorie TOTAL ____

Optional Records.
Blood Sugar:
Blood Pressure:
Other:
TODAY'S Calorie TOTAL ____

Optional Records.
Blood Sugar:
Blood Pressure:
Other:
TODAY'S Calorie TOTAL ____

Optional Records.
Blood Sugar:
Blood Pressure:
Other:
TODAY'S Calorie TOTAL ____

"Weigh yourself in your 'birthday suit' ONE time every morning at the same time."

"Use the 'Optional Records' section if you need to track other health issues"

Section Four: **Tracking Your Weight Loss**

Going, Going... Gone!

Now we are going to **track your progress** and record and graph your weight loss.

You will find **copies** of all of the **forms** shown in the pages that follow. You will be using them to transfer your results from your daily menu planners and daily keep track of your **vanishing 'pounds and inches.'**

"Now we are going to track your progress and record and graph your weight loss."

"...transfer your results from your daily menu planners and daily keep track of your vanishing 'pounds and inches."

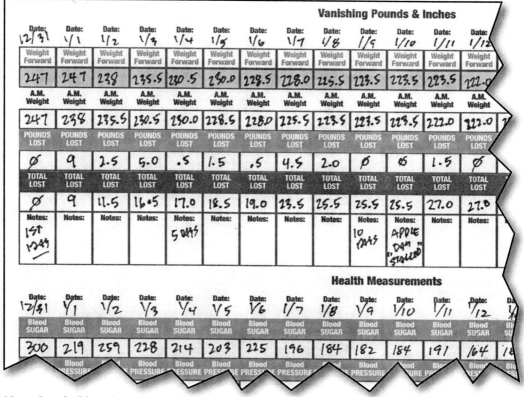

Keeping it Simple.

You will note that the **form above** covers 20 days, or as the doctor would put it, one 'course' of HCG treatment.

"...it is really simple and takes but a few minutes to complete."

Don't be intimidated by this form, it is really **simple** and takes but a few **minutes** to complete. Just start at the upper left corner. Fill in the date. Under **'Weight Forward'** write today's weight. Moving straight down fill in **'A.M. Weight.'** Note: On your **first** day, those first two **weight numbers** will be **the same**.

Okay, move straight down to **'Pounds Lost'** and then **'Total Lost,'** once again on the first day, both of these will be the same... that would be zero. Keep going down and make any **'Notes'** and add any personal **'Health Measurements'** or **'RX Records'** (you know... prescriptions) that **you and your doctor** have determined are needed on a **daily basis**. That's all there is to it.

On the **second day** the previous days **'A.M. Weight'** moves **over and up** to the **'Weight Forward'** box. Then write in **today's weight** and **subtract** to get the **'Pounds Lost.'** To arrive at the **'Total Lost'** you simply **add** todays **'Pounds Lost'** to yesterdays **'Total Lost'** which will give you the **'fun number'**...your pounds lost. Also don't forget to record the other **measurements** you are tracking.

Section Four: Tracking Your Weight Loss

Your 'Poof it's Gone' Chart.

One of the funest and most **exciting things** you can do to keep **motivated** and **on course** is to transfer your pounds & inches **numbers,** to the chart **shown below.**

If you are doing it right you will most likely experience what all of the HCG Alums experience. That would be **dramatic** and rapid **weight loss,** followed by, of course, disappearing **inches.** A slight lag between the two is perfectly normal.

As I have shared before, **I lost 22 pounds** in the first **7 days,** so brace yourself.

"One of the funnest and most exciting things you can do to keep motivated..."

"...dramatic and rapid weight loss, followed by, of course, disappearing inches..."

Color in the POUNDS as You Lose Them!

These are the Actual Pounds I lost on the HCG + 500 Calorie Diet Phase

The Proof is in the 'Poofing.'

Here is **how to use** this 'Poof' recap chart.

"...each box represents one pound lost..."

Look in the center and you will see a series of **numbers** from **'-1'** to **'-47'** that is the number of accumulative **pounds** you have **lost.** That figure comes from the **'Total Lost'** box on your **'Vanishing Pounds & Inches'** form that we just covered.

On this form, you just **color** in the number of vertical boxes, **each box** represents **one pound lost,** to graphically show your pounds lost. It's that fun and simple.

Be sure to **record the dates** carefully, of course, and utilize the other optional parts of the form to track your **measurements, medical conditions** or **medications.**

 ISBN 978-0-9800641-7-9

Vanishing Pounds & Inches

Date:	Date:	Date:	Date:	Date:	Date:	Date:	Date:	Date:	Date:	Date:	Date:	Date:	Date:	Date:	Date:	Date:	Date:	Date:	Date:
Weight Forward	Weight Forward	Weight Forward	Weight Forward	Weight Forward	Weight Forward	Weight Forward	Weight Forward	Weight Forward	Weight Forward	Weight Forward	Weight Forward	Weight Forward	Weight Forward	Weight Forward	Weight Forward	Weight Forward	Weight Forward	Weight Forward	Weight Forward
A.M. Weight	A.M. Weight	A.M. Weight	A.M. Weight	A.M. Weight	A.M. Weight	A.M. Weight	A.M. Weight	A.M. Weight	A.M. Weight	A.M. Weight	A.M. Weight	A.M. Weight	A.M. Weight	A.M. Weight	A.M. Weight	A.M. Weight	A.M. Weight	A.M. Weight	A.M. Weight
POUNDS LOST	POUNDS LOST	POUNDS LOST	POUNDS LOST	POUNDS LOST	POUNDS LOST	POUNDS LOST	POUNDS LOST	POUNDS LOST	POUNDS LOST	POUNDS LOST	POUNDS LOST	POUNDS LOST	POUNDS LOST	POUNDS LOST	POUNDS LOST	POUNDS LOST	POUNDS LOST	POUNDS LOST	POUNDS LOST
TOTAL LOST	TOTAL LOST	TOTAL LOST	TOTAL LOST	TOTAL LOST	TOTAL LOST	TOTAL LOST	TOTAL LOST	TOTAL LOST	TOTAL LOST	TOTAL LOST	TOTAL LOST	TOTAL LOST	TOTAL LOST	TOTAL LOST	TOTAL LOST	TOTAL LOST	TOTAL LOST	TOTAL LOST	TOTAL LOST
Notes:	Notes:	Notes:	Notes:	Notes:	Notes:	Notes:	Notes:	Notes:	Notes:	Notes:	Notes:	Notes:	Notes:	Notes:	Notes:	Notes:	Notes:	Notes:	Notes:

Optional Health Measurements

Date:	Date:	Date:	Date:	Date:	Date:	Date:	Date:	Date:	Date:	Date:	Date:	Date:	Date:	Date:	Date:	Date:	Date:	Date:	Date:
Blood SUGAR	Blood SUGAR	Blood SUGAR	Blood SUGAR	Blood SUGAR	Blood SUGAR	Blood SUGAR	Blood SUGAR	Blood SUGAR	Blood SUGAR	Blood SUGAR	Blood SUGAR	Blood SUGAR	Blood SUGAR	Blood SUGAR	Blood SUGAR	Blood SUGAR	Blood SUGAR	Blood SUGAR	Blood SUGAR
Blood PRESSURE	Blood PRESSURE	Blood PRESSURE	Blood PRESSURE	Blood PRESSURE	Blood PRESSURE	Blood PRESSURE	Blood PRESSURE	Blood PRESSURE	Blood PRESSURE	Blood PRESSURE	Blood PRESSURE	Blood PRESSURE	Blood PRESSURE	Blood PRESSURE	Blood PRESSURE	Blood PRESSURE	Blood PRESSURE	Blood PRESSURE	Blood PRESSURE
RX Records	RX Records	RX Records	RX Records	RX Records	RX Records	RX Records	RX Records	RX Records	RX Records	RX Records	RX Records	RX Records	RX Records	RX Records	RX Records	RX Records	RX Records	RX Records	RX Records

ISBN 978-0-9800641-7-9

Vanishing Pounds & Inches

Date:	Date:	Date:	Date:	Date:	Date:	Date:	Date:	Date:	Date:	Date:	Date:	Date:	Date:	Date:	Date:
Weight Forward															
A.M. Weight															
POUNDS LOST															
TOTAL LOST															
Notes:															

Optional Health Measurements

Date:	Date:	Date:	Date:	Date:	Date:	Date:	Date:	Date:	Date:	Date:	Date:	Date:
Blood SUGAR												
Blood PRESSURE												
RX Records												

ISBN 978-0-9800641-7-9

Vanishing Pounds & Inches

Date:	Date:	Date:	Date:	Date:	Date:	Date:	Date:	Date:	Date:	Date:	Date:	Date:	Date:	Date:	Date:	Date:	Date:	Date:	Date:
Weight Forward	Weight Forward	Weight Forward	Weight Forward	Weight Forward	Weight Forward	Weight Forward	Weight Forward	Weight Forward	Weight Forward	Weight Forward	Weight Forward	Weight Forward	Weight Forward	Weight Forward	Weight Forward	Weight Forward	Weight Forward	Weight Forward	Weight Forward
A.M. Weight	A.M. Weight	A.M. Weight	A.M. Weight	A.M. Weight	A.M. Weight	A.M. Weight	A.M. Weight	A.M. Weight	A.M. Weight	A.M. Weight	A.M. Weight	A.M. Weight	A.M. Weight	A.M. Weight	A.M. Weight	A.M. Weight	A.M. Weight	A.M. Weight	A.M. Weight
POUNDS LOST	POUNDS LOST	POUNDS LOST	POUNDS LOST	POUNDS LOST	POUNDS LOST	POUNDS LOST	POUNDS LOST	POUNDS LOST	POUNDS LOST	POUNDS LOST	POUNDS LOST	POUNDS LOST	POUNDS LOST	POUNDS LOST	POUNDS LOST	POUNDS LOST	POUNDS LOST	POUNDS LOST	POUNDS LOST
TOTAL LOST	TOTAL LOST	TOTAL LOST	TOTAL LOST	TOTAL LOST	TOTAL LOST	TOTAL LOST	TOTAL LOST	TOTAL LOST	TOTAL LOST	TOTAL LOST	TOTAL LOST	TOTAL LOST	TOTAL LOST	TOTAL LOST	TOTAL LOST	TOTAL LOST	TOTAL LOST	TOTAL LOST	TOTAL LOST
Notes:	Notes:	Notes:	Notes:	Notes:	Notes:	Notes:	Notes:	Notes:	Notes:	Notes:	Notes:	Notes:	Notes:	Notes:	Notes:	Notes:	Notes:	Notes:	Notes:

Optional Health Measurements

Date:	Date:	Date:	Date:	Date:	Date:	Date:	Date:	Date:	Date:	Date:	Date:	Date:	Date:	Date:	Date:	Date:	Date:	Date:	Date:
Blood SUGAR	Blood SUGAR	Blood SUGAR	Blood SUGAR	Blood SUGAR	Blood SUGAR	Blood SUGAR	Blood SUGAR	Blood SUGAR	Blood SUGAR	Blood SUGAR	Blood SUGAR	Blood SUGAR	Blood SUGAR	Blood SUGAR	Blood SUGAR	Blood SUGAR	Blood SUGAR	Blood SUGAR	Blood SUGAR
Blood PRESSURE	Blood PRESSURE	Blood PRESSURE	Blood PRESSURE	Blood PRESSURE	Blood PRESSURE	Blood PRESSURE	Blood PRESSURE	Blood PRESSURE	Blood PRESSURE	Blood PRESSURE	Blood PRESSURE	Blood PRESSURE	Blood PRESSURE	Blood PRESSURE	Blood PRESSURE	Blood PRESSURE	Blood PRESSURE	Blood PRESSURE	Blood PRESSURE

RX Records	RX Records	RX Records	RX Records	RX Records	RX Records	RX Records	RX Records	RX Records	RX Records	RX Records	RX Records	RX Records	RX Records	RX Records	RX Records	RX Records	RX Records	RX Records	RX Records

					Month																		
Month					**Day**																		
Day																							
Location					-1																		
R. Wrist					-2																		
L. Wrist					-3																		
Waist					-4																		
Fat 'Roll' A					-5																		
Fat 'Roll' B					-6																		
Upper Chest					-7																		
Midriff					-8																		
Hips					-9																		
R. Thigh					-10																		
L. Thigh					-11																		
R. Knee					-12																		
L. Knee					-13																		
R. Calf					-14																		
L. Calf					-15																		
L. Knee					-16																		
L. Knee					-17																		
					-18																		
					-19																		
TOTALS					-20																		
Notes:					-21																		
					-22																		
					-23																		
Health Measurements & Check-ups					-24																		
Item/Date					-25																		
B. Sugar					-26																		
B. Pressure					-27																		
B. Pressure					-28																		
					-29																		
					-30																		
					-31																		
					-32																		
					-33																		
					-34																		
RX/Quit Date					-35																		
					-36																		
					-37																		
					-38																		
					-39																		
					-40																		
					-41																		
					-42																		
					-43																		
					-44																		
					-45																		
					-46																		
					-47																		

Your Very Own "Poof it's gone!" CHART

Month					Month																					
Day					**Day**																					
Location					-1																					
R. Wrist					-2																					
L. Wrist					-3																					
Waist					-4																					
Fat 'Roll' A					-5																					
Fat 'Roll' B					-6																					
Upper Chest					-7																					
Midriff					-8																					
Hips					-9																					
R. Thigh					-10																					
L. Thigh					-11																					
R. Knee					-12																					
L. Knee					-13																					
R. Calf					-14																					
L. Calf					-15																					
L. Knee					-16																					
L. Knee					-17																					
					-18																					
					-19																					
TOTALS					-20																					
Notes:					-21																					
					-22																					
					-23																					
Health Measurements & Check-ups					-24																					
Item/Date					-25																					
B. Sugar					-26																					
B. Pressure					-27																					
B. Pressure					-28																					
					-29																					
					-30																					
					-31																					
					-32																					
					-33																					
					-34																					
RX/Quit Date					-35																					
					-36																					
					-37																					
					-38																					
					-39																					
					-40																					
					-41																					
					-42																					
					-43																					
					-44																					
					-45																					
					-46																					
					-47																					

Your Very Own
"Poof it's gone!"
CHART

HCG + 500 CALORIES

BASIC RECIPES

BASIC RECIPES · HCG + 500

ISBN 978-0-9800641-7-9

Section Four: **HCG + 500 Calorie Tested Recipes**

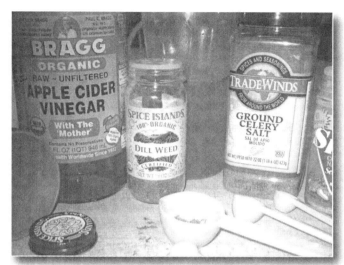

Shown here are some of the things you will need to make your 'Mom in a Bottle' dressing a success.

Taste Tested Tips & Techniques

Fresh fruit will normally be a part of the **basic salad recipes** which adds some **natural sweetness** and flavor.

You can use **any variety of apple** so experiment until you find a few favorites. **Refrigerate apples** as soon as you get them home. Always store at **42-45 degrees** to preserve the quality and crispness of your apples.

'Mom in a Bottle' Apple Cider Vinegar All Purpose Dressing

Summary of this Tested Recipe:

Organic Apple Cider Vinegar dressing is your friend. This all purpose **salad dressing** will be a stalwart in your **tool kit**. Take some time and **perfect it**.

You will come to love it.

Adding your favorite **sugarless seasonings** to personalize it, is part of the fun.

I like the tartness of the **Apple Cider Vinegar,** so I skipped the sweetener. Do some tasting and you will find the right combination for your taste buds.

Keep in mind as you eat the allowed foods and flavorings, **your taste buds will sharpen** and you may want to adjust the formula.

When you are done it will taste just like **mom** made it.

Write down **your ingredients** and put the top on it and put it in the fridge. Always better when chilled.

You can use this dressing on **salads** and on **meats**. It adds very few **calories** and all of the benefits of natural **'organic vinegar.'**

What You Will Need:

Apple Cider Vinegar
Organic Raw & Unfiltered
with the 'Mother' in the bottle.

Purified Water
Filtered or bottled

Sugarless Seasonings
Check the ingredients on the label for any hidden sugars. Your preference. See suggestions below.

Mixing Bottle with cap
Used to mix the ingredients and shake and store for use on your salads.

Keep Refrigerated

The Recipe:

4 oz. Apple Cider Vinegar
Organic Raw & Unfiltered
with the 'Mother' in it.

8 oz. Pure Water

Seasonings Choices
1/2 tsp Celery Salt
1/4 tsp Onion salt
Dash of Dill Weed
Dash of Garlic Salt

Optional:
Natural sweetener such as Agave Nectar or Liquid Stevia.

Fresh 'Organic' Lemon

Here's What You Do:

Measure and add **water** and **vinegar** to your **mixing bottle**. Start adding the **basic seasonings** in the amounts suggested and then **season to your taste** buds. Be sure to shake well. The dressing will be a little tart by itself. If it is too tart, you may like the **optional sweeteners**. I prefer the Agave, some like Stevia instead. Go slow. These natural sweeteners are **very strong** compared to sugar. A little goes a long way. Fresh **Lemon juice** is optional.

The flavors of the **lettuce** and **apples** and **meat** in the finished salad will modify it. It's best to taste test after application to your salad recipe. Cap it up and chill. There you have it... **'Mom in a Bottle.'** Shake well before **each** use.

2 oz = 10 Calories

Section Four: HCG + 500 Calorie Tested Recipes

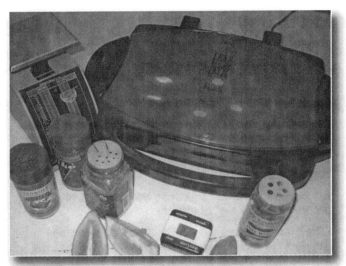

Shown above is my favorite model of the George Foreman Grill. Works very well. I prefer the model with the removable parts. Makes cleaning much simpler and easier.

Getting 'Mean' with Protein.

Summary:

Since you obviously are **trimming and weighing** your meat while **raw,** it follows that some type of cooking is required and there are a few choices to make.

This page **covers the basics** of preparing your **PROTEIN** focusing on 'Preparation' and 'Cooking Methods' Covered are **barbecue, broiling, baking** or using the infamous George Foreman "...lean... mean... grillin'...machine."

We'll look at the pluses and minuses of these methods. Plus some **tips** and **techniques.**

This should help with preparing your chosen source of protein, and achieving the necessary variety and rotation needed for your **HCG + 500 Calorie** menu plan.

Here are some guidelines.

What You Will Need:

Gas Grill barbecue
Cooking in **batches** is recommended. A gas grill is more convenient and pollution free. Much **easier to control** the temperature consistently. A Built in thermometer is a big plus.

Oven or Broiler Oven
Use your oven for baking and broiling. A broiler oven will work as well.

George Foreman Grill
Lots of different models. I like the larger ones with the **removable** cooking plates for ease of cleaning. A good investment.

Your 'Sugar Free' Seasonings
Go on a shopping expedition and stock up on **sugar free seasoning** for meat. You can find them everywhere. Some are labeled **'Poultry or Steak Seasoning'** some are flavored for general use.

Portable Kitchen Timer
One you can carry around is great.

Your Imagination
Try a few different seasoning and cooking methods, until you find the ones you like. A little **seasoning** and **marinating** before cooking, just takes a little bit of **planning and time** and will add to your **enjoyment** and **satisfaction.**

Taste Tested Tips & Techniques

BEEF and VEAL: Cooking Suggestions

Shopping Tip:

Save some money by checking the meat department in your store for items **marked for quick sale.** These are meats that are near their 'sell by' dates. They are perfectly fine if you take them home and either **cook or freeze immediately.**

Best Preparation:

A good approach is to **do batches** of meat. I like to cut, trim and weigh them right after I bring them home. Then **I cook a batch** or **freeze** in marked bags. Once you get the habit you will **always have a supply** of meat ready.

If frozen, thaw. **Trim all visible fat** and if you haven't done this already, weigh RAW, cutting pieces to 3.75 oz.

Pre season and/or marinate 3-4 hours before cooking. Wash your hands and utensials carefully before and after. A great approach is to sprinkle on your beef seasoning and then **massage it** into the meat a little.

For a simple marinade that tastes great and is safe, use your **'Mom in a bottle' dressing.** The vinegar is a natural meat tenderizer so don't over marinate.

Best Cooking Methods.

Number One: Barbecue on the **gas grill** on medium **low heat** (250 degrees temperature on your BBQ) purchase a **cheap but loud** timer. Start out setting it for **5 minutes.** Warm the BBQ for 5 minutes. When the alarm goes off, **reset it** as you add your seasoned and marinated meat to the grill. **Turn every 5 minutes,** each time setting the timer before you turn the meat. Repeat until you get the desired doneness you like, trying not to over cook. **Be patient.**

Number Two: 'George Foreman Grill.' Most don't have a heat setting, just on or off. The **only control is time.** Use your timer and try different settings. Start with 2 minutes. Different cuts of meat are a little different, so once again **cook in batches and experiment** until you find the right setting for you. Write down the answer for next time. You will be able to easily **repeat the results.**

Section Four: HCG + 500 Calorie Tested Recipes

Taste Tested Tips & Techniques

CHICKEN: Cooking Suggestions

Shopping Tip:

Buy frozen, skinless chicken breasts. You can find these in the 'all natural' and sometimes 'organic' variety. They are processed and dipped in water and **flash frozen**. So they are just as fresh, maybe fresher than the 'fresh' ones in the meat case. Price is reasonable as there is **very little waste**.

Best Preparation:

Once again, a good approach is to **do batches**. Start with **two chicken breasts**, which allowing for rotation, will give you enough (4 servings) for 2 days. I find that the frozen chicken breasts as they come in the package, are about the right weight when **cut in half** and trimmed.

Place a batch of **frozen chicken breasts** in a pan to thaw. I like to sprinkle them with a good 'poultry seasoning'.

Partially thaw.

Just thaw enough so that you can trim and cut them, but they are **still frozen enough** to **retain some moisture** from the freezing process. **Trim all visible fat** and weigh RAW **cutting pieces to 3.75 oz.**
Always wash your hands and utensials carefully.

Best Cooking Methods.

Number One: You should start **barbecueing** on the **gas grill** on **medium low heat** (250 degrees) **before** completely thawed. This will result in **moister and more tender** chicken.

Use your cheap but loud timer. Start out setting it for 5 minutes. Warm the BBQ for 5 minutes. When the alarm goes off, **restart it as you add** your seasoned chicken breasts to the grill. Turn every 5 minutes, each time setting the timer **before you turn** the meat. (Less chance that you will forget and over-cook!) Repeat until you get the desired doneness you like, **trying not to over cook.** Be patient.

The best barbecuing secret? Go slow!

Number Two: Because of the slight tendency of the 'George Foreman Grill' to dry chicken out, **baking** is my next recommendation **for great chicken** results.

Best Preparation:

The same preparation as above **except** completely thaw the chicken pieces before baking. Once again, a good approach is to **do batches**. Baked chicken keeps well.

Use a **fresh baking dish** that is large enough to **avoid stacking** the chicken pieces. Line the bottom of the dish with fresh **baby spinach leaves**. A good heavy layer. Place seasoned chicken and top each piece with a thin slice of **fresh lemon**.

Cover with tin foil and bake at 375 for about 40 minutes. Ovens do vary, so **test** the chicken **the first time** to get the exact time, for the doneness you prefer. Write it down.

Number Three: Use the 'George Forman Grill,' much the same way that you did the beef grilling. With **a little practice** you will easily figure out the amount of time you need. Be careful to **avoid drying out** the chicken, by overcooking .

The great thing about this grill is, it removes excess fat. Not a lot of that in a properly trimmed chicken breast. Once you do figure out the correct time, it is **very repeatable** with George's 'lean mean grillin' machine. Write down your **cooking time**.

CHICKEN EGGS: Protein in a shell

Best Preparation.

Eggs are a source of **protein** you can utilize and said to be one of nature's most complete foods.

Studies have been done that would indicate that eggs as a source of **cholesterol** related problems is way **overblown**. If you are over concerned about cholesterol, a good optional approach is to use two egg whites for each egg yolk.

I think where eggs get a bad rap is from the most prevalent **method of preparation**... that would be 'fried'... don't!

Best Cooking Methods.

Cook your eggs by **boiling** or **poaching** and you are getting the beneficial inputs from eggs and minimizing the negative.

SEAFOOD: Low Fat Fish, Shellfish, Shrimp

Best Preparation.

Be careful to use very fresh or frozen varieties of the species listed in the HCG + 500 Seafood charts.
Seafood is available in many fresh frozen varieties or you may have the opportunity to catch it your self.

Best Cooking Methods.

Seafood can be cooked the same as chicken, that would be **barbecue**, **bake** and **grill** and **in addition steamed**.

Seafood **cooks very quickly**, so once again some **testing** and experimenting when cooking it the first time, will serve you well.

Watch out for **sugar** in the seafood seasoning and sauces.

Seafood is a category of food that **can cause** your weight loss to **stall** or **diminish**. If you have that problem look at your menu records, if you suspect the seafood is the problem **cut back** or **eliminate** it for the **HCG + 500 Calorie** phase of treatment.

SUMMARY: Have Some Fun!

It helps to **keep your perspective**. You can do this! It is just a such **a short time** in your life and staying focused and giving it your best effort will really pay off with what can be **life changing** results and **very quickly** the pounds and inches will just melt away and it will all be worth it!

Just go for it!

Section Four: HCG + 500 Calorie Tested Recipes

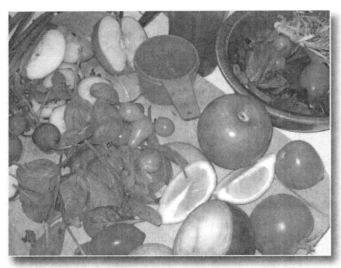

The 'Apple ChickenSalad' shown here was created using the 'Go-To Green Salad' and adding crisp Gala Apples and skinless trimmed & grilled chicken breast and the 'Mom in a Bottle' Dressing recipe you just learned. Low Calories and very tasty.

The Basic 'Go-To' Green Salad.

Summary of this Tested Recipe:

A basic green salad will normally be the foundation for a number of variations of basic salad recipes.

This recipe **covers the basics** and some additions to achieve the necessary variety and rotation needed for your **HCG + 500 Calorie** menu plan.

Making good **fresh and nutritious** salads with some **eye appeal** goes a long way toward keeping things **simple** and on **target**. Under 250 calories and filling.

You can use **any variety of apple** so experiment until you find a few favorites. Just changing from a sweet to a tart apple, not to mention **the color it adds**, can change the **flavor** and **taste** so you don't get bored.

Refrigerate apples as soon as you get them home. Store at 42-45 degrees for maximum crispy life.

What You Will Need:

Green Lettuce Mix
Organic & Fresh & Clean!
You can find a variety of these and they are normally reasonably priced and carefully washed and packaged

Baby Spinach Leaves
Rotation of your vegetables is a key. So you can easily substitute this vegetable choice for the lettuce.

Fresh & Crisp Apples
Any variety will work. Each one adds a variation of taste and eye appeal and even crispness. Have fun... experiment!

Fresh 'Organic' Lemon
You can eat a lemon everyday. I like to squeeze fresh lemon juice on my salads just before eating.

A bonus is the **lemon juice** keeps the apples from turning brown.

Your Choice of Protein
Use a variety, remembering to rotate the protein type, watch the Calories here!

Your 'Mom in a Bottle' Homemade Dressing
Experiment a little and customize this to your taste buds. Best to taste **test after applying** to your salad.

The Recipe:

2 Cups of Lettuce or Baby Spinach
Organic is best. Chop slightly just before preparing to help release the flavor. (2 cups 42/22 Calories)

1 Medium Apple (Your Choice)
Organic is best. Core & Chop to bite sized. (70 Calories)

1/4 Cup 'Mom in a Bottle' Apple Cider Vinegar Dressing
Your custom Mix (2 oz. 10 Calories)

Optional Additions:
3.75 oz. Protein of Choice
Fat Free Chicken (85 Calories)
Low Fat Beef (185 Calories)
Low Fat Fish (80-110 Calories)

Juice 1/4 Fresh Lemon (optional)
0 Calories)

Taste Tested Tips & Techniques

Take a **handful of lettuce** or **baby leaf spinach** and roll it up and cut just before you are ready to eat your salad. This **releases the flavor** of the greenery. Can you smell it?

It is best to mix just the amount of salad **you are going to eat** and make it up fresh each time. Just takes a few minutes and it will taste **fresher, crispier and more flavorful**.

Here's What You Do:

Lightly chop **lettuce** or **baby spinach**. Place in a shallow bowl or dish. Add your choice of **cut up apples** and your choice of **meat** with all visible fat removed.

Shake up your **'Mom in a Bottle'** homemade dressing and **add to salad**. Toss well and enjoy.

(165-240 Calories Depending on protein choice)

Section Four: **HCG + 500 Calorie Tested Recipes**

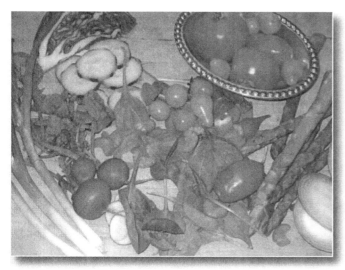

The 'Veggie Team'

Your 'Veggie Team' Substitutes

Summary: How to use your 'bench.'

You have your meat cooked.
You have your 'Mom in a Bottle' dressing
You have fixed a 'go to' green salad.

Now what?

Let's review. Making good **fresh and nutritious** salads with some **eye appeal** goes a long way toward keeping things simple and on target and **under 250 calories.**

You can use **any variety of apple.** Want to know how to get the rest of the **veggie team** involved, to change the flavor and taste, so you don't get bored?

Check out the ideas below.

Taste Tested Tips & Techniques

ASPARAGUS (4 oz. = 25 Calories)

Cooked: Steam or boil.
Use as a main vegetable instead of salad.
'Mom in a Bottle' Dressing is great with this.

CABBAGE (1 cup = 27 Calories)

Raw: cut like 'cole slaw' add chopped apple and 'Mom in a Bottle' Dressing
Cooked: Bake with chicken or veal

CELERY (1 cup = 17 Calories)

Salad: Chop and mix with chopped apple for a fresh crunchy, crunchy salad. Make dressing add 1/4 cup pureed cottage cheese (58 Calories) and 'Mom in a Bottle.'
By the stalk: Stuff with cotttage cheese and a dash of dill weed. Great for a snack.

CUCUMBERS (1 cup = 16 Calories)

Raw: Slice and put in a bowl of Mom in a Bottle dressing. Chill well. You can also make a cucumber and apple salad.

ONIONS (1 small = 29 Calories)

Grilled: The 'George Foreman Grill' works great.
You can add these to the grill at the same time as your steak and grill together. Adds a nice flavor. Changes the cooking.
Baked: Bake in the oven (350 for 75 minutes) and eat with seasoning, salt and pepper or dressing.

RED RADISHES (1 cup = 30 Calories)

Raw: I like to slice these very thin and salt and eat like potato chips. Filling and very low Calorie.

SPINACH, RAW/COOKED (1 cup = 11/41 Calories)

Raw: Use as a salad substitute.
Cooked: Bake with your chicken.
Steamed: Use as your main vegetable

TOMATOES, Cherry (1 cup = 27 Calories)

Raw: A great low Calorie snack, that is oozing with nutrients.
Cooked: Puree and add to organic beef or chicken broth. Makes a nice soup. Great on a cold day.

TOMATOES, Medium (1 medium = 35 Calories)

Raw: A great low Calorie snack, that is oozing with nutrients.
Cooked: Puree and add to organic beef or chicken broth. Makes a nice soup. Great on a cold day.

NOTE: Tomatoes are a potential weight loss staller!

Where's the LETTUCE?

The Lettuce is a star!

See the 'Go to Green Salad'

Section Four: **HCG + 500 Calorie Tested Recipes**

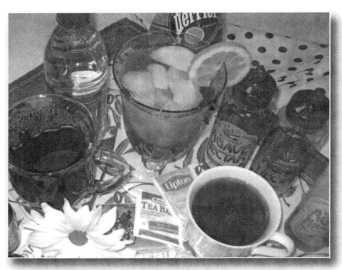

Water... Water... Everywhere? What else to drink?

Water, Water...Not Everywhere?

Summary: 'Variations on a Theme'

No Limit on Approved Drinks.

Let's review what is **approved** by the good doctor **without restrictions:**

- **All types of Coffees & Teas**
- **Pure Mineral Water**
- **Pure Fresh Water**
- **Daily Fresh Squeezed Lemon Juice**

Your fluid intake should be **at least 68 oz.** a day.

Drinking hot or cold liquids does help **curb** and **control** your **appetite.**

Check out the ideas below.

Taste Tested Tips & Techniques

HOT DRINKS:

HOT COFFEE:
Organic whenever possible, decaf or the regular kind.

Additives:
Natural sweeteners, Stevia is actually available in lots of flavors. They have a four flavor small portable assortment you can carry around. Sorry, only 1 tablespoon of milk a day.

Coffee is a **'diuretic.'** Doctor talk for frequent bladder emptying. So be sure to drink plenty of other liquids.

HOT TEAS:
Organic whenever possible, decaf or the regular kind. Teas also claim to have other desirable benefits. Check the labels.

Additives:
Natural sweeteners, Stevia is actually available in lots of Flavors. They have a four flavor small portable assortment you can carry around. Sorry, only 1 tablespoon of milk a day.

Tea is an **'acid.'** Tannic acid to be precise. Some find it upsetting on an empty stomach. Also a **'diuretic.'** So be sure to drink plenty of other liquids.

HOT CHOCOLATE:
Actually made with hot water and 'chocolate' flavored Stevia.

Additives:
Sorry, only 1 tablespoon of milk a day.

Some find this good and add some other flavored Stevia to customize it. Helps if you are a chocolate craver. I am not a Stevia lover, but start with about five drops and experiment a little.

COLD DRINKS:

ICED COFFEE:
Organic whenever possible, decaf or the regular kind. A nice refreshing drink on a hot summer day!

Additives:
Natural sweeteners, Stevia is actually available in lots of flavors. They have a four flavor small portable assortment you can carry around. Sorry, only 1 tablespoon of milk a day.

Coffee is a **'diuretic.'** Doctor talk for frequent bladder emptying. So be sure to drink plenty of other liquids.

ICED TEA:
Organic whenever possible, decaf or the regular kind. 'Sun tea' is my favorite way of brewing. Refrigerate until nice and frosty.

Additives:
Natural sweeteners, Stevia is actually is available in lots of flavors. They have a four flavor small portable assortment you can carry around. Sorry, only 1 tablespoon of milk a day.

Tea is an **'acid.'** Tannic acid to be precise. Some find it upsetting on an empty stomach. Also a **'diuretic.'** So be sure to drink plenty of other liquids.

ICED COLD LEMONADE:
Fresh squeezed Organic Lemon juice added to water or mineral water. Refrigerate until nice and frosty.

Additives:
Natural sweeteners, Stevia is available in fruit flavors. Agave Nectar, is now flavored, as well. You can make a fake strawberry lemonade. Later you add real strawberries as you finish your **HCG + 500 Calorie** phase.

Section Five:

'Listen to the Good Doctor.'

"What I have to say is, in essence, the views distilled out of 40 years of grappling with the fundamental problems of obesity, its causes, its symptoms, and its very nature."

Dr. A.T.W. Simeons

Defeat OBESITY...Forever!

The HCG Assisted 500 Calorie Weight Loss Cure

Section Five: **Reference: Dr. Simeons Manuscript**

Introduction and Comments.

A.T.W. Simeons in my opinion, was to **obesity and its control**, what Einstein was to Quantum Physics. He was **relentless**, patient, resourceful and blessed with a brilliant and inquiring mind. Because he refused to accept the **commonly held misconceptions** about obesity, and labored for much of his life in relative obscurity with one goal in mind... to help all mankind, those of us who struggle with obesity, can rejoice!

What follows is an 'illuminated' reproduction of his commonly available **original short manuscript**. I have tried to present his work in an **easily referenced** and **highlighted** form in the hopes that you would be drawn to **read and study** it, and thus fully come to embrace and appreciate his discoveries. If you do you will be the better for it. With apologies to Doctor Simeons, I have added a **Table of Content**s and a few **simple graphic diagrams** and **flow charts** meant to **visually enhance**, not detract from **his fine work**.

Pounds & Inches

A NEW APPROACH TO OBESITY

By: Dr. A.T.W. Simeons

Salvator Mundi International Hospital 00152 - Rome Viale Mura Gianicolensi, 77

Summary of Contents

Section Five: **Reference: Dr. Simeons Manuscript**

Section Five: **Reference: Dr. Simeons Manuscript**

Section Five:

Foreword by Doctor Simeons:

"...a method of treatment which has grown out of theoretical considerations based on clinical observations."

"...overeating is the result of the disorder, not it's cause..."

"...more and more facts seemed to fit snugly into the new framework..."

This book discusses a new interpretation of the nature of obesity, and while it does not advocate yet another This book discusses a **new interpretation of the nature of obesity**, and while it does not advocate another fancy slimming diet it does describe a method of treatment which has grown out of theoretical considerations based on clinical observation.

What I have to say is an essence of views distilled out of forty years of grappling with the fundamental problems of obesity, its causes, its symptoms, and its very nature. In these many years of specialized work thousands of cases have passed through my hands and were carefully studied. Every new theory, every new method, every promising lead was considered, experimentally screened and critically evaluated as soon as it became known. But invariably the results were disappointing and lacking in uniformity.

I felt that we were merely nibbling at the fringe of a great problem, as, indeed, do most serious students of overweight. We have grown pretty sure that the tendency to accumulate abnormal fat is a very definite metabolic disorder, much as is, for instance, diabetes. Yet the localization and the nature of this disorder remained a mystery. Every new approach seemed to lead into a blind alley, and though patients were told that they are fat because they eat too much, we believed that this is neither the whole truth nor the last word in the matter.

Refusing to be side-tracked by an all too facile interpretation of obesity, I have always held that overeating is the result of the disorder, not its cause, and that we can make little headway until we can build for ourselves some sort of theoretical structure with which to explain the condition. Whether such a structure represents the truth is not important at this moment. What it must do is to give us an intellectually satisfying interpretation of what is happening in the obese body. It must also be able to withstand the onslaught of all hitherto known clinical facts and furnish a hard background against which the results of treatment can be accurately assessed.

To me this requirement seems basic, and it has always been the center of my interest. In dealing with obese patients it became a habit to register and order every clinical experience as if it were an odd looking piece of a jig-saw puzzle. And then, as in a jig saw puzzle, little clusters of fragments began to form, though they seemed to fit in nowhere. As the years passed these clusters grew bigger and started to amalgamate until, about sixteen years ago, a complete picture became dimly discernible. This picture was, and still is, dotted with gaps for which I cannot find the pieces, but I do now feel that a theoretical structure is visible as a whole.

With mounting experience, more and more facts seemed to fit snugly into the new framework, and when then a treatment based on such speculations showed consistently satisfactory results, I was sure that some practical advance had been made, regardless of whether the theoretical interpretation of these results is correct or not.

The clinical results of the new treatment have been published in scientific journal [1] and these reports have been generally well received by the profession, but the very nature of a scientific article does not permit the full presentation of new theoretical concepts nor is there room to discuss the finer points of technique and the reasons for observing them.

Section Five:

Foreword by Doctor Simeons:

"...experience through the many trials and errors which I have long since overcome."

"Only then can there be intelligent cooperation between physician and patient."

"I shall be unashamedly authoritative and avoid all the hedging and tentativeness."

During the 16 years that have elapsed since I first published my findings, I have had many hundreds of inquiries from research institutes, doctors and patients. Hitherto I could only refer those interested to my scientific papers, though I realized that these did not contain sufficient information to enable doctors to conduct the new treatment satisfactorily. Those who tried were obliged to gain their own experience through the many trials and errors which I have long since overcome.

Doctors from all over the world have come to Italy to study the method, first hand in my clinic in the Salvator Mundi International Hospital in Rome. For some of them the time they could spare has been too short to get a full grasp of the technique, and in any case the number of those whom I have been able to meet personally is small compared with the many requests for further detailed information which keep coming in. I have tried to keep up with these demands by correspondence, but the volume of this work has become unmanageable and that is one excuse for writing this book.

In dealing with a disorder in which the patient must take an active part in the treatment, it is, I believe, essential that he or she have an understanding of what is being done and why. Only then can there be intelligent cooperation between physician and patient. In order to avoid writing two books, one for the physician and another for the patient - a prospect which would probably have resulted in no book at all - I have tried to meet the requirements of both in a single book. This is a rather difficult enterprise in which I may not have succeeded. The expert will grumble about long-windedness while the lay-reader may occasionally have to look up an unfamiliar word in the **glossary** provided for him.

To make the text more readable I shall be unashamedly authoritative and avoid all the hedging and tentativeness with which it is customary to express new scientific concepts grown out of clinical experience and not as yet confirmed by clear-cut laboratory experiments. Thus, when I make what reads like a factual statement, the professional reader may have to translate into: clinical experience seems to suggest that such and such an observation might be tentatively explained by such and such a working hypothesis, requiring a vast amount of further research before the hypothesis can be considered a valid theory. If we can from the outset establish this as a mutually accepted convention, I hope to avoid being accused of speculative exuberance.

Section Five:　　**The Nature of Obesity**

"...an abnormal functioning of some part of the body..."

Obesity a Disorder

As a basis for our discussion we postulate that obesity in all its many forms is due to an abnormal functioning of some part of the body and that every ounce of abnormally accumulated fat is always the result of the same disorder of certain regulatory mechanisms.

Persons suffering from this particular disorder will get fat regardless of whether they eat excessively, normally or less than normal. A person who is free of the disorder will never get fat, even if he frequently overeats.

Those in whom the disorder is severe will accumulate fat very rapidly, those in whom it is moderate will gradually increase in weight and those in whom it is mild may be able to keep their excess weight stationary for long periods. In all these cases a loss of weight brought about by dieting, treatments with thyroid, appetite-reducing drugs, laxatives, violent exercise, massage, baths, etc., is only temporary and will be rapidly regained as soon as the reducing regimen is relaxed. The reason is simply that none of these measures corrects the basic disorder.

While there are great variations in the severity of obesity, we shall consider all the different forms in both sexes and at all ages as always being due to the same disorder. Variations in form would then be partly a matter of degree, partly an inherited bodily constitution and partly the result of a secondary involvement of endocrine glands such as the pituitary, the thyroid, the adrenals or the sex glands. On the other hand, we postulate that no deficiency of any of these glands can ever directly produce the common disorder known as obesity.

"...it follows that a treatment aimed at curing the disorder must be equally effective in both sexes, at all ages and in all forms of obesity."

If this reasoning is correct, it follows that a treatment aimed at curing the disorder must be equally effective in both sexes, at all ages and in all forms of obesity. Unless this is so, we are entitled to harbor grave doubts as to whether a given treatment corrects the underlying disorder. Moreover, any claim that the disorder has been corrected must be substantiated by the ability of the patient to eat normally of any food he pleases without regaining abnormal fat after treatment. Only if these conditions are fulfilled can we legitimately speak of curing obesity rather than of reducing weight.

Our problem thus presents itself as an enquiry into the localization and the nature of the disorder which leads to obesity. The history of this enquiry is a long series of high hopes and bitter disappointments.

The History of Obesity

There was a time, not so long ago, when obesity was considered a sign of health and prosperity in man and of beauty, amorousness and fecundity in women. This attitude probably dates back to Neolithic times, about 8000 years ago; when for the first time in the history of culture, man began to own property, domestic animals, arable land, houses, pottery and metal tools. Before that, with the possible exception of some races such as the Hottentots, obesity was almost non-existent, as it still is in all wild animals and most primitive races.

Today obesity is extremely common among all civilized races, because a disposition to the disorder can be inherited. Wherever abnormal fat was regarded as an asset,

"...the trend still lingers on."

sexual selection tended to propagate the trait. It is only in very recent times that manifest obesity has lost some of its allure, though the cult of the outsize bust - always a sign of latent obesity - shows that the trend still lingers on.

The Significance of Regular Meals

In the early Neolithic times another change took place which may well account for the fact that today nearly all inherited dispositions sooner or later develop into manifest obesity. This change was the institution of regular meals. In pre-Neolithic times, man ate only when he was hungry and only as much as he required to still the pangs of hunger. Moreover, much of his food was raw and all of it was unrefined. He roasted his meat, but he did not boil it, as he had no pots, and what little he may have grubbed from the Earth and picked from the trees, he ate as he went along.

The whole structure of man's omnivorous digestive tract is, like that of an ape, rat or pig, adjusted to the continual nibbling of tidbits. It is not suited to occasional gorging as is, for instance, the intestine of the carnivorous cat family. Thus the institution of regular meals, particularly of food rendered rapidly assimilable, placed a great burden on modern man's ability to cope with large quantities of food suddenly pouring into his system from the intestinal tract.

The institution of regular meals meant that man had to eat more than his body required at the moment of eating so as to tide him over until the next meal. Food rendered easily digestible suddenly flooded his body with nourishment of which he was in no need at the moment. Somehow, somewhere this surplus had to be stored.

Three Kinds of Fat

"...a great burden on modern man's ability to cope with large quantities of food suddenly pouring into his system..."

In the human body we can distinguish three kinds of fat. The **first** is the **structural fat** which fills the gaps between various organs, a sort of packing material. Structural fat also performs such important functions as bedding the kidneys in soft elastic tissue, protecting the coronary arteries and keeping the skin smooth and taut. It also provides the springy cushion of hard fat under the bones of the feet, without which we would be unable to walk.

The **second type of fat** is a **normal reserve of fuel** upon which the body can freely draw when the nutritional income from the intestinal tract is insufficient to meet the demand. Such normal reserves are localized all over the body. Fat is a substance which packs the highest caloric value into the smallest space so that normal reserves of fuel for muscular activity and the maintenance of body temperature can be most economically stored in this form. Both these types of fat, structural and reserve, are normal, and even if the body stocks them to capacity this can never be called obesity.

But there is **a third type of fat which is entirely abnormal**. It is the accumulation of such fat, and of such fat only, from which the overweight patient suffers. This abnormal fat is also a potential reserve of fuel, but unlike the normal reserves it is not available to the body in a nutritional emergency. It is, so to speak, locked away in a fixed deposit and is not kept in a current account **[2]**, as are the normal reserves.

When an obese patient tries to reduce by starving himself, he will first lose his normal fat reserves. When these are exhausted he begins to burn up structural fat, and only

"...obese patients complain that when they diet they lose the wrong fat."

as a last resort will the body yield its abnormal reserves, though by that time the patient usually feels so weak and hungry that the diet is abandoned. It is just for this reason that obese patients complain that when they diet they lose the wrong fat. They feel famished and tired and their face becomes drawn and haggard, but their belly, hips, thighs and upper arms show little improvement. The fat they have come to detest stays on and the fat they need to cover their bones gets less and less. Their skin wrinkles and they look old and miserable. And that is one of the most frustrating and depressing experiences a human being can have.

Injustice to the Obese

When then obese patients are accused of cheating, gluttony, lack of will power, greed and sexual complexes, the strong become indignant and decide that modern medicine is a fraud and its representatives fools, while the weak just give up the struggle in despair. In either case the result is the same: a further gain in weight, resignation to an abominable fate and the resolution at least to live tolerably the short span allotted to them - a fig for doctors and insurance companies.

"Obese patients only feel physically well as long as they are stationary or gaining weight."

Obese patients only feel physically well as long as they are stationary or gaining weight. They may feel guilty, owing to the lethargy and indolence always associated with obesity. They may feel ashamed of what they have been led to believe is a lack of control. They may feel horrified by the appearance of their nude body and the tightness of their clothes. But they have a primitive feeling of animal content which turns to misery and suffering as soon as they make a resolute attempt to reduce. For this there are sound reasons.

In the first place, more caloric energy is required to keep a large body at a certain temperature than to heat a small body. Secondly the muscular effort of moving a heavy body is greater than in the case of a light body. The muscular effort consumes Calories which must be provided by food. Thus, all other factors being equal, a fat person requires more food than a lean one. One might therefore reason that if a fat person eats only the additional food his body requires he should be able to keep his weight stationary. Yet every physician who has studied obese patients under rigorously controlled conditions knows that this is not true.

Many obese patients actually gain weight on a diet which is calorically deficient for their basic needs. There must thus be some other mechanism at work.

"There must thus be some other mechanism at work."

Glandular Theories

At one time it was thought that this mechanism might be concerned with the sex glands. Such a connection was suggested by the fact that many juvenile obese patients show an under-development of the sex organs. The middle-age spread in men and the tendency of many women to put on weight in the menopause seemed to indicate a causal connection between diminishing sex function and overweight. Yet, when highly active sex hormones became available, it was found that their administration had no effect whatsoever on obesity. The sex glands could therefore not be the seat of the disorder.

Section Five: **The Nature of Obesity**

The Thyroid Gland

When it was discovered that the thyroid gland controls the rate at which body-fuel is consumed, it was thought that by administering thyroid gland to obese patients their abnormal fat deposits could be burned up more rapidly. This too proved to be entirely disappointing, because as we now know, these abnormal deposits take no part in the body's energy-turnover - they are inaccessibly locked away. Thyroid medication merely forces the body to consume its normal fat reserves, which are already depleted in obese patients, and then to break down structurally essential fat without touching the abnormal deposits. In this way a patient may be brought to the brink of starvation in spite of having a hundred pounds of fat to spare. Thus any weight loss brought about by thyroid medication is always at the expense of fat of which the body is in dire need.

"Thyroid medication merely forces the body to consume its normal fat reserves..."

While the majority of obese patients have a perfectly normal thyroid gland and some even have an overactive thyroid, one also occasionally sees a case with a real thyroid deficiency. In such cases, treatment with thyroid brings about a small loss of weight, but this is not due to the loss of any abnormal fat. It is entirely the result of the elimination of a mucoid substance, called myxedema, which the body accumulates when there is a marked primary thyroid deficiency. Moreover, patients suffering only from a severe lack of thyroid hormone never become obese in the true sense. Possibly also the observation that normal persons - though not the obese - lose weight rapidly when their thyroid becomes overactive may have contributed to the false notion that thyroid deficiency and obesity are connected. Much misunderstanding about the supposed role of the thyroid gland in obesity is still met with, and it is now really high time that thyroid preparations be once and for all struck off the list of remedies for obesity. This is particularly so because giving thyroid gland to an obese patient whose thyroid is either normal or overactive, besides being useless, is decidedly dangerous.

The Pituitary Gland

"...not a single one or any combination of such factors proved to be of any value in the treatment of obesity."

The next gland to be falsely incriminated was the anterior lobe of the pituitary, or hypophysis. This most important gland lies well protected in a bony capsule at the base of the skull. It has a vast number of functions in the body, among which is the regulation of all the other important endocrine glands. The fact that various signs of anterior pituitary deficiency are often associated with obesity raised the hope that the seat of the disorder might be in this gland. But although a large number of pituitary hormones have been isolated and many extracts of the gland prepared, not a single one or any combination of such factors proved to be of any value in the treatment of obesity. Quite recently, however, a fat-mobilizing factor has been found in pituitary glands, but it is still too early to say whether this factor is destined to play a role in the treatment of obesity.

The Adrenals

Recently, a long series of brilliant discoveries concerning the working of the adrenal or suprarenal glands, small bodies which sit atop the kidneys, have created tremendous interest. This interest also turned to the problem of obesity when it was discovered that a condition which in some respects resembles a severe case of obesity - the so called Cushing's Syndrome - was caused by a glandular new-growth of the adrenals or by their excessive stimulation with ACTH, which is the pituitary hormone governing the activity of the outer rind or cortex of the adrenals.

Section Five: **The Nature of Obesity**

"...this knowledge furnished no practical means of treating obesity..."

When we learned that an abnormal stimulation of the adrenal cortex could produce signs that resemble true obesity, this knowledge furnished no practical means of treating obesity by decreasing the activity of the adrenal cortex. There is no evidence to suggest that in obesity there is any excess of adrenocortical activity; in fact, all the evidence points to the contrary. There seems to be rather a lack of adrenocortical function and a decrease in the secretion of ACTH from the anterior pituitary lobe.[3]

So here again our search for the mechanism which produces obesity led us into a blind alley. Recently, many students of obesity have reverted to the nihilistic attitude that obesity is caused simply by overeating and that it can only be cured by under eating.

The 'Diencephalon' or 'Hypothalamus.'

"...the complex operation of storing and issuing fuel to the body might also be controlled by the diencephalon..."

For those of us who refused to be discouraged there remained one slight hope. Buried deep down in the massive human brain there is a part which we have in common with all vertebrate animals the so-called diencephalon. It is a very primitive part of the brain and has in man been almost smothered by the huge masses of nervous tissue with which we think, reason and voluntarily move our body. The diencephalon is the part from which the central nervous system controls all the automatic animal functions of the body, such as breathing, the heart beat, digestion, sleep, sex, the urinary system, the autonomous or vegetative nervous system and via the pituitary the whole interplay of the endocrine glands.

It was therefore not unreasonable to suppose that the complex operation of storing and issuing fuel to the body might also be controlled by the diencephalon. It has long been known that the content of sugar - another form of fuel - in the blood depends on a certain nervous center in the diencephalon. When this center is destroyed in laboratory animals, they develop a condition rather similar to human stable diabetes. It has also long been known that the destruction of another diencephalic center produces a voracious appetite and a rapid gain in weight in animals which never get fat spontaneously.

The Fat-bank

"...a point may be reached which goes beyond the diencephalon's banking capacity..."

Assuming that in man such a center controlling the movement of fat does exist, its function would have to be much like that of a bank. When the body assimilates from the intestinal tract more fuel than it needs at the moment, this surplus is deposited in what may be compared with a current account. Out of this account it can always be withdrawn as required. All normal fat reserves are in such a current account, and it is probable that a diencephalic center manages the deposits and withdrawals.

When now, for reasons which will be discussed later, the deposits grow rapidly while small withdrawals become more frequent, a point may be reached which goes beyond the diencephalon's banking capacity. Just as a banker might suggest to a wealthy client that instead of accumulating a large and unmanageable current account he should invest his surplus capital, the body appears to establish a fixed deposit into which all surplus funds go but from which they can no longer be withdrawn by the procedure used in a current account. In this way the diencephalic "fat-bank" frees itself from all work which goes beyond its normal banking capacity. The onset of obesity dates from the moment the diencephalon adopts this labor-saving ruse. Once a fixed deposit has been established the normal fat reserves are held at a minimum,

Section Five: **Three Basic Causes of Obesity**

while every available surplus is locked away in the fixed deposit and is therefore taken out of normal circulation.

Three Basic Causes of Obesity:

(1) The Inherited Factor

"...the fat-banking capacity is abnormally low from birth."

Assuming that there is a limit to the diencephalon's fat banking capacity, it follows that there are three basic ways in which obesity can become manifest. The first is that the fat-banking capacity is abnormally low from birth. Such a congenitally low diencephalic capacity would then represent the inherited factor in obesity. When this abnormal trait is markedly present, obesity will develop at an early age in spite of normal feeding; this could explain why among brothers and sisters eating the same food at the same table some become obese and others do not.

(2) Other Diencephalic Disorders

"...the lowering of a previously normal fat-banking capacity..."

The second way in which obesity can become established is the lowering of a previously normal fat-banking capacity owing to some other diencephalic disorder. It seems to be a general rule that when one of the many diencephalic centers is particularly overtaxed; it tries to increase its capacity at the expense of other centers.

In the menopause and after castration the hormones previously produced in the sex-glands no longer circulate in the body. In the presence of normally functioning sex-glands their hormones act as a brake on the secretion of the sex-gland stimulating hormones of the anterior pituitary.

When this brake is removed the anterior pituitary enormously increases its output of these sex-gland stimulating hormones, though they are now no longer effective. In the absence of any response from the non-functioning or missing sex glands, there is nothing to stop the anterior pituitary from producing more and more of these hormones. This situation causes an excessive strain on the diencephalic center which controls the function of the anterior pituitary. In order to cope with this additional burden the center appears to draw more and more energy away from other centers, such as those concerned with emotional stability, the blood circulation (hot flushes) and other autonomous nervous regulations, particularly also from the not so vitally important fat-bank.

"...the fat-banking capacity is reduced to the point at which it is forced to establish a 'fixed deposit' and thus initiate the disorder we call obesity."

The so-called stable type of diabetes heavily involves the diencephalic blood sugar regulating center. The diencephalon tries to meet this abnormal load by switching energy destined for the fat bank over to the sugar-regulating center, with the result that the fat-banking capacity is reduced to the point at which it is forced to establish a fixed deposit and thus initiate the disorder we call obesity. In this case one would have to consider the diabetes the primary cause of the obesity, but it is also possible that the process is reversed in the sense that a deficient or overworked fat-center draws energy from the sugar-center, in which case the obesity would be the cause of that type of diabetes in which the pancreas is not primarily involved. Finally, it is conceivable that in Cushing's syndrome those symptoms which resemble obesity are entirely due to the withdrawal of energy from the diencephalic fat-bank in order to make it available to the highly disturbed center which governs the anterior pituitary adrenocortical system.

Section Five: **Three Basic Causes of Obesity**

"...its insurgence obviously has nothing to do with..."

Whether obesity is caused by a marked inherited deficiency of the fat-center or by some entirely different diencephalic regulatory disorder, its insurgence obviously has nothing to do with overeating and in either case obesity is certain to develop regardless of dietary restrictions. In these cases any enforced food deficit is made up from essential fat reserves and normal structural fat, much to the disadvantage of the patient's general health.

(3) The Exhaustion of the Fat-bank

But there is still a third way in which obesity can become established, and that is when a presumably normal fat-center is suddenly -- the emphasis is on suddenly -- called upon to deal with an enormous influx of food far in excess of momentary requirements. At first glance it does seem that here we have a straight-forward case of overeating being responsible for obesity, but on further analysis it soon becomes clear that the relation of cause and effect is not so simple. In the first place we are merely assuming that the capacity of the fat center is normal while it is possible and even probable that only persons who have some inherited trait in this direction can become obese merely by overeating.

Secondly, in many of these cases the amount of food eaten remains the same and it is only the consumption of fuel which is suddenly decreased, as when an athlete is confined to bed for many weeks with a broken bone or when a man leading a highly active life is suddenly tied to his desk in an office and to television at home. Similarly, when a person, grown up in a cold climate, is transferred to a tropical country and continues to eat as before, he may develop obesity because in the heat far less fuel is required to maintain the normal body temperature.

"...the rush of incoming fuel which occurs at every meal may eventually overpower the diecenphalic regulatory mechanisms and thus lead to obesity."

When a person suffers a long period of privation, be it due to chronic illness, poverty, famine or the exigencies of war, his diencephalic regulations adjust themselves to some extent to the low food intake. When then suddenly these conditions change and he is free to eat all the food he wants, this is liable to overwhelm his fat-regulating center. During the last war [4] about 6000 grossly underfed Polish refugees who had spent harrowing years in Russia were transferred to a camp in India where they were well housed, given normal British army rations and some cash to buy a few extras. Within about three months, 85% were suffering from obesity.

In a person eating coarse and unrefined food, the digestion is slow and only a little nourishment at a time is assimilated from the intestinal tract. When such a person is suddenly able to obtain highly refined foods such as sugar, white flour, butter and oil these are so rapidly digested and assimilated that the rush of incoming fuel which occurs at every meal may eventually overpower the diecenphalic regulatory mechanisms and thus lead to obesity. This is commonly seen in the poor man who suddenly becomes rich enough to buy the more expensive refined foods, though his total caloric intake remains the same or is even less than before.

ISBN 978-0-9800641-7-9

Section Five: **Psychological Aspects**

Much has been written about the psychological aspects of obesity. Among its many functions the diencephalon is also the seat of our primitive animal instincts, and just as in an emergency it can switch energy from one center to another, so it seems to be able to transfer pressure from one instinct to another. Thus, a lonely and unhappy person deprived of all emotional comfort and of all instinct gratification except the stilling of hunger and thirst can use these as outlets for pent up instinct pressure and so develop obesity. Yet once that has happened, no amount of psychotherapy or analysis, happiness, company or the gratification of other instincts will correct the condition.

Compulsive Eating

"No end of injustice is done to obese patients by accusing them of compulsive eating..."

No end of injustice is done to obese patients by accusing them of compulsive eating, which is a form of diverted sex gratification. Most obese patients do not suffer from compulsive eating; they suffer genuine hunger - real, gnawing, torturing hunger - which has nothing whatever to do with compulsive eating. Even their sudden desire for sweets is merely the result of the experience that sweets, pastries and alcohol will most rapidly of all foods allay the pangs of hunger. This has nothing to do with diverted instincts.

On the other hand, compulsive eating does occur in some obese patients, particularly in girls in their late teens or early twenties. Compulsive eating differs fundamentally from the obese patient's greater need for food. It comes on in attacks and is never associated with real hunger, a fact which is readily admitted by the patients. They only feel a feral desire to stuff. Two pounds of chocolates may be devoured in a few minutes; cold, greasy food from the refrigerator, stale bread, leftovers on stacked plates, almost anything edible is crammed down with terrifying speed and ferocity.

"Patients suffering from real compulsive eating are comparatively rare."

I have occasionally been able to watch such an attack without the patient's knowledge, and it is a frightening, ugly spectacle to behold, even if one does realize that mechanisms entirely beyond the patient's control are at work. A careful enquiry into what may have brought on such an attack almost invariably reveals that it is preceded by a strong unresolved sex-stimulation, the higher centers of the brain having blocked primitive diencephalic instinct gratification. The pressure is then let off through another primitive channel, which is oral gratification. In my experience the only thing that will cure this condition is uninhibited sex, a therapeutic procedure which is hardly ever feasible, for if it were, the patient would have adopted it without professional prompting, nor would this in any way correct the associated obesity. It would only raise new and often greater problems if used as a therapeutic measure.

Patients suffering from real compulsive eating are comparatively rare. In my practice they constitute about 1-2%. Treating them for obesity is a heartrending job. They do perfectly well between attacks, but a single bout occurring while under treatment may annul several weeks of therapy. Little wonder that such patients become discouraged. In these cases I have found that psychotherapy may make the patient fully understand the mechanism, but it does nothing to stop it. Perhaps society's growing sexual permissiveness will make compulsive eating even rarer.

Whether a patient is really suffering from compulsive eating or not is hard to decide before treatment because many obese patients think that their desire for food -- to them unmotivated -- is due to compulsive eating, while all the time it is merely a greater

Section Five:	Psychological Aspects

need for food. The only way to find out is to treat such patients. Those that suffer from real compulsive eating continue to have such attacks, while those who are not compulsive eaters never get an attack during treatment.

Reluctance to Lose Weight

"Some patients are deeply attached to their fat and cannot bear the thought of losing it."

Some patients are deeply attached to their fat and cannot bear the thought of losing it. If they are intelligent, popular and successful in spite of their handicap, this is a source of pride. Some fat girls look upon their condition as a safeguard against erotic involvements, of which they are afraid. They work out a pattern of life in which their obesity plays a determining role and then become reluctant to upset this pattern and face a new kind of life which will be entirely different after their figure has become normal and often very attractive. They fear that people will like them - or be jealous - on account of their figure rather than be attracted by their intelligence or character only. Some have a feeling that reducing means giving up an almost cherished and intimate part of themselves. In many of these cases psychotherapy can be helpful, as it enables these patients to see the whole situation in the full light of consciousness. An affectionate attachment to abnormal fat is usually seen in patients who became obese in childhood, but this is not necessarily so.

In all other cases the best psychotherapy can do in the usual treatment of obesity is to render the burden of hunger and never-ending dietary restrictions slightly more tolerable. Patients who have successfully established an erotic transfer to their psychiatrist are often better able to bear their suffering as a secret labor of love.

"...a large number of ways in which obesity can be initiated..."

There are thus a large number of ways in which obesity can be initiated, though the disorder itself is always due to the same mechanism, an inadequacy of the diencephalic fat-center and the laying down of abnormally fixed fat deposits in abnormal places. This means that once obesity has become established, it can no more be cured by eliminating those factors which brought it on than a fire can be extinguished by removing the cause of the conflagration. Thus a discussion of the various ways in which obesity can become established is useful from a preventative point of view, but it has no bearing on the treatment of the established condition. The elimination of factors which are clearly hastening the course of the disorder may slow down its progress or even halt it, but they can never correct it.

Not by Weight Alone

"Weight alone is not a satisfactory criterion by which to judge whether a person is suffering from the disorder we call obesity..."

Weight alone is not a satisfactory criterion by which to judge whether a person is suffering from the disorder we call obesity or not. Every physician is familiar with the sylphlike lady who enters the consulting room and declares emphatically that she is getting horribly fat and wishes to reduce. Many an honest and sympathetic physician at once concludes that he is dealing with a "nut." If he is busy he will give her short shrift, but if he has time he will weigh her and show her tables to prove that she is actually underweight.

I have never yet seen or heard of such a lady being convinced by either procedure. The reason is that in my experience the lady is nearly always right and the doctor wrong. When such a patient is carefully examined one finds many signs of potential obesity, which is just about to become manifest as overweight. The patient distinctly

Section Five: **Signs and Symptoms of Obesity**

feels that something is wrong with her, that a subtle change is taking place in her body, and this alarms her.

There are a number of signs and symptoms which are characteristic of obesity. In manifest obesity many and often all these signs and symptoms are present. In latent or just beginning cases some are always found, and it should be a rule that if two or more of the bodily signs are present, the case must be regarded as one that needs immediate help.

"There are a number of signs and symptoms which are characteristic of obesity."

Signs and Symptoms of Obesity

The bodily signs may be divided into such as have developed before puberty, indicating a strong inherited factor, and those which develop at the onset of manifest disorder. Early signs are a disproportionately large size of the two upper front teeth, the first incisor, or a dimple on both sides of the sacral bone just above the buttocks. When the arms are outstretched with the palms upward, the forearms appear sharply angled outward from the upper arms. The same applies to the lower extremities. The patient cannot bring his feet together without the knees overlapping; he is, in fact, knock-kneed.

"The beginning accumulation of abnormal fat..."

The beginning accumulation of abnormal fat shows as a little pad just below the nape of the neck, colloquially known as the Duchess' Hump. There is a triangular fatty bulge in front of the armpit when the arm is held against the body. When the skin is stretched by fat rapidly accumulating under it, it may split in the lower layers. When large and fresh, such tears are purple, but later they are transformed into white scar-tissue. Such striation, as it is called, commonly occurs on the abdomen of women during pregnancy, but in obesity it is frequently found on the breasts, the hips and occasionally on the shoulders. In many cases striation is so fine that the small white lines are only just visible. They are always a sure sign of obesity, and though this may be slight at the time of examination such patients can usually remember a period in their childhood when they were excessively chubby.

"...remember that any number of these signs may be present in persons whose weight is statistically normal..."

Another typical sign is a pad of fat on the insides of the knees, a spot where normal fat reserves are never stored. There may be a fold of skin over the pubic area and another fold may stretch round both sides of the chest, where a loose roll of fat can be picked up between two fingers. In the male an excessive accumulation of fat in the breasts is always indicative, while in the female the breast is usually, but not necessarily, large. Obviously excessive fat on the abdomen, the hips, thighs, upper arms, chin and shoulders are characteristic, and it is important to remember that any number of these signs may be present in persons whose weight is statistically normal; particularly if they are dieting on their own with iron determination.

Common clinical symptoms which are indicative only in their association and in the frame of the whole clinical picture are: frequent headaches, rheumatic pains without detectable bony abnormality; a feeling of laziness and lethargy, often both physical and mental and frequently associated with insomnia, the patients saying that all they want is to rest; the frightening feeling of being famished and sometimes weak with hunger two to three hours after a hearty meal and an irresistible yearning for sweets and starchy food which often overcomes the patient quite suddenly and is sometimes substituted by a desire for alcohol; constipation and a spastic or irritable colon are unusually common among the obese, and so are menstrual disorders.

   Signs and Symptoms of Obesity

"I have yet to see a patient who continues to complain..."

Returning once more to our sylphlike lady, we can say that a combination of some of these symptoms with a few of the typical bodily signs is sufficient evidence to take her case seriously. A human figure, male or female, can only be judged in the nude; any opinion based on the dressed appearance can be quite fantastically wide off the mark, and I feel myself driven to the conclusion that apart from frankly psychotic patients such as cases of anorexia nervosa; a morbid weight fixation does not exist. I have yet to see a patient who continues to complain after the figure has been rendered normal by adequate treatment.

The Emaciated Lady

I remember the case of a lady who was escorted into my consulting room while I was telephoning. She sat down in front of my desk, and when I looked up to greet her I saw the typical picture of advanced emaciation. Her dry skin hung loosely over the bones of her face, her neck was scrawny and collarbones and ribs stuck out from deep hollows. I immediately thought of cancer and decided to which of my colleagues at the hospital I would refer her. Indeed, I felt a little annoyed that my assistant had not explained to her that her case did not fall under my specialty. In answer to my query as to what I could do for her, she replied that she wanted to reduce. I tried to hide my surprise, but she must have noted a fleeting expression, for she smiled and said "I know that you think I'm mad, but just wait." With that she rose and came round to my side of the desk. Jutting out from a tiny waist she had enormous hips and thighs.

"...the abnormal fat on her hips was transferred to the rest of her body..."

By using a technique which will presently be described, the abnormal fat on her hips was transferred to the rest of her body which had been emaciated by months of very severe dieting. At the end of a treatment lasting five weeks, she, a small woman, had lost 8 inches round her hips, while her face looked fresh and florid, the ribs were no longer visible and her weight was the same to the ounce as it had been at the first consultation.

Fat but not Obese

"...it is also possible for a person to be statistically overweight without suffering from obesity."

While a person who is statistically underweight may still be suffering from the disorder which causes obesity, it is also possible for a person to be statistically overweight without suffering from obesity. For such persons weight is no problem, as they can gain or lose at will and experience no difficulty in reducing their caloric intake. They are masters of their weight, which the obese are not. Moreover, their excess fat shows no preference for certain typical regions of the body, as does the fat in all cases of obesity. Thus, the decision whether a borderline case is really suffering from obesity or not cannot be made merely by consulting weight tables.

Section Five: **The Treatment of Obesity**

If obesity is always due to one very specific diencephalic deficiency, it follows that the only way to cure it is to correct this deficiency. At first this seemed an utterly hopeless undertaking. The greatest obstacle was that one could hardly hope to correct an inherited trait localized deep inside the brain, and while we did possess a number of drugs whose point of action was believed to be in the diencephalon, none of them had the slightest effect on the fat-center. There was not even a pointer showing a direction in which pharmacological research could move to find a drug that had such a specific action. The closest approach were the appetite-reducing drugs - the amphetamines----- but these cured nothing.

A Curious Observation

"...appetite reducing drugs, the amphetamines but these cured nothing."

Mulling over this depressing situation, I remembered a rather curious observation made many years ago in India. At that time we knew very little about the function of the diencephalon, and my interest centered round the pituitary gland. Froehlich had described cases of extreme obesity and sexual underdevelopment in youths suffering from a new growth of the anterior pituitary lobe, producing what then became known as Froehlich's disease. However, it was very soon discovered that the identical syndrome, though running a less fulminating course, was quite common in patients whose pituitary gland was perfectly normal. These are the so-called "fat boys" with long, slender hands, breasts any flat-chested maiden would be proud to posses, large hips, buttocks and thighs with striation, knock-knees and underdeveloped genitals, often with undescended testicles.

It also became known that in these cases the sex organs could he developed by giving the patients injections of a substance extracted from the urine of pregnant women, it having been shown that when this substance was injected into sexually immature rats it made them precociously mature. The amount of substance which produced this effect in one rat was called one International Unit, and the purified extract was accordingly called "Human Chorionic Gonadotrophin" whereby chorionic signifies that it is produced in the placenta and gonadotropin that its action is sex gland directed.

"...a substance extracted from the urine of pregnant women..."

The usual way of treating "fat boys" with underdeveloped genitals is to inject several hundred International Units twice a week. **Human Chorionic Gonadotrophin** which we shall henceforth simply call **HCG** is expensive and as "fat boys" are fairly common among Indians I tried to establish the smallest effective dose. In the course of this study three interesting things emerged.

The first was that when fresh pregnancy-urine from the female ward was given in quantities of about 300 cc. by retention enema, as good results could be obtained as by injecting the pure substance. The second was that small daily doses appeared to be just as effective as much larger ones given twice a week. Thirdly, and that is the observation that concerns us here, when such patients were given small daily doses they seemed to lose their ravenous appetite though they neither gained nor lost weight. Strangely enough however, their shape did change. Though they were not restricted in diet, there was a distinct decrease in the circumference of their hips.

Section Five: **The Treatment of Obesity**

Fat on the Move

"...it occurred to me that the change in shape could only be explained by a movement of fat away from abnormal deposits..."

Remembering this, it occurred to me that the change in shape could only be explained by a movement of fat away from abnormal deposits on the hips, and if that were so there was just a chance that while such fat was in transition it might be available to the body as fuel. This was easy to find out, as in that case, fat on the move would be able to replace food. It should then he possible to keep a "fat boy" on a severely restricted diet without a feeling of hunger, in spite of a rapid loss of weight. When I tried this in typical cases of Froehlich's syndrome, I found that as long as such patients were given small daily doses of HCG they could comfortably go about their usual occupations on a diet of only 500 Calories daily and lose an average of about one pound per day. It was also perfectly evident that only abnormal fat was being consumed, as there were no signs of any depletion of normal fat. Their skin remained fresh and turgid, and gradually their figures became entirely normal, nor did the daily administration of HCG appear to have any side-effects other than beneficial.

From this point it was a small step to try the same method in all other forms of obesity. It took a few hundred cases to establish beyond reasonable doubt that the mechanism operates in exactly the same way and seemingly without exception in every case of obesity. I found that, though most patients were treated in the outpatients department, gross dietary errors rarely occurred. On the contrary, most patients complained that the two meals of 250 Calories each were more than they could manage, as they continually had a feeling of just having had a large meal.

"...given small daily doses of HCG they could comfortably go about their usual occupations on a diet of only 500 Calories daily and lose an average of about one pound per day."

Pregnancy and Obesity

Once this trail was opened, further observations seemed to fall into line. It is, for instance, well known that during pregnancy an obese woman can very easily lose weight. She can drastically reduce her diet without feeling hunger or discomfort and lose weight without in any way harming the child in her womb. It is also surprising to what extent a woman can suffer from pregnancy-vomiting without coming to any real harm.

Pregnancy is an obese woman's one great chance to reduce her excess weight. That she so rarely makes use of this opportunity is due to the erroneous notion, usually fostered by her elder relations, that she now has "two mouths to feed" and must "keep up her strength for the coming event. All modern obstetricians know that this is nonsense and that the more superfluous fat is lost the less difficult will be the confinement, though some still hesitate to prescribe a diet sufficiently low in Calories to bring about a drastic reduction.

"...during pregnancy, an obese woman, can very easily lose weight."

A woman may gain weight during pregnancy, but she never becomes obese in the strict sense of the word. Under the influence of the HCG which circulates in enormous quantities in her body during pregnancy, her diencephalic banking capacity seems to be unlimited, and abnormal fixed deposits are never formed. At confinement [5] she is suddenly deprived of HCG, and her diencephalic fat-center reverts to its normal capacity. It is only then that the abnormally accumulated fat is locked away again in a fixed deposit. From that moment on she is suffering from obesity and is subject to all its consequences.

Section Five: **The Treatment of Obesity**

"...only during pregnancy that fixed fat deposits can be transferred back into the normal current account and freely drawn upon to make up for any nutritional deficit."

Pregnancy seems to be the only normal human condition in which the diencephalic fat-banking capacity is unlimited. It is only during pregnancy that fixed fat deposits can be transferred back into the normal current account and freely drawn upon to make up for any nutritional deficit. During pregnancy, every ounce of reserve fat is placed at the disposal of the growing fetus. Were this not so, an obese woman, whose normal reserves are already depleted, would have the greatest difficulties in bringing her pregnancy to full term. There is considerable evidence to suggest that it is the HCG produced in large quantities in the placenta which brings about this diencephalic change.

Though we may be able to increase the dieneephalic fat banking capacity by injecting HCG, this does not in itself affect the weight, just as transferring monetary funds from a fixed deposit into a current account does not make a man any poorer; to become poorer it is also necessary that he freely spends the money which thus becomes available. In pregnancy the needs of the growing embryo take care of this to some extent, but in the treatment of obesity there is no embryo, and so a very severe dietary restriction must take its place for the duration of treatment.

"... obese patients under treatment with HCG never feel hungry..."

Only when the fat which is in transit under the effect of HCG is actually consumed can more fat be withdrawn from the fixed deposits. In pregnancy it would be most undesirable if the fetus were offered ample food only when there is a high influx from the intestinal tract. Ideal nutritional conditions for the fetus can only be achieved when the mother's blood is continually saturated with food, regardless of whether she eats or not, as otherwise a period of starvation might hamper the steady growth of the embryo. It seems that HCG brings about this continual saturation of the blood, which is the reason why obese patients under treatment with HCG never feel hungry in spite of their drastically reduced food intake.

Shown at right:

Illustration H

An added flow chart illustration of the protocol discovered by Dr. Simeons

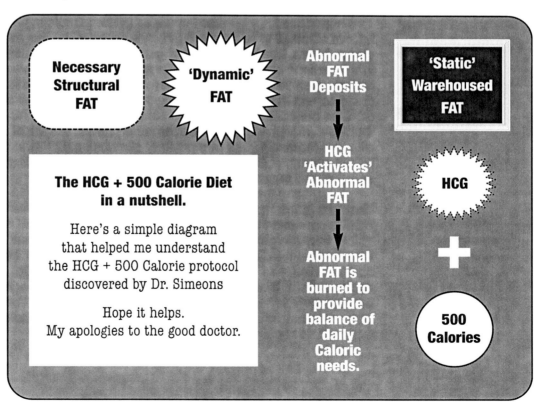

Necessary Structural FAT

'Dynamic' FAT

Abnormal FAT Deposits

'Static' Warehoused FAT

HCG 'Activates' Abnormal FAT

HCG

The HCG + 500 Calorie Diet in a nutshell.

Here's a simple diagram that helped me understand the HCG + 500 Calorie protocol discovered by Dr. Simeons

Hope it helps.
My apologies to the good doctor.

Abnormal FAT is burned to provide balance of daily Caloric needs.

+

500 Calories

Section Five: **Human Chorionic Gonadotropin (HCG)**

"HCG is never found in the human body except during pregnancy..."

HCG is never found in the human body except during pregnancy and in those rare cases in which a residue of placental tissue continues to grow in the womb in what is known as a chorionic epithelioma. It is never found in the male. The human type of chorionic gonadotrophin is found only during the pregnancy of women and the great apes. It is produced in enormous quantities, so that during certain phases of her pregnancy a woman may excrete as much as one million International Units per day in her urine - enough to render a million infantile rats precociously mature. Other mammals make use of a different hormone, which can be extracted from their blood serum but not from their urine. Their placenta differs in this and other respects from that of man and the great apes. This animal chorionic gonadotrophin is much less rapidly broken down in the human body than HCG, and it is also less suitable for the treatment of obesity.

"...acts exclusively at a diencephalic level and there brings about a considerable increase in the functional capacity..."

As often happens in medicine, much confusion has been caused by giving HCG its name before its true mode of action was understood. It has been explained that gonadotrophin literally means a sex-gland directed substance or hormone, and this is quite misleading. It dates from the early days when it was first found that HCG is able to render infantile sex glands mature, whereby it was entirely overlooked that it has no stimulating effect whatsoever on normally developed and normally functioning sex-glands. No amount of HCG is ever able to increase a normal sex function; it can only improve an abnormal one and in the young hasten the onset of puberty. However, this is no direct effect. HCG acts exclusively at a diencephalic level and there brings about a considerable increase in the functional capacity of all those centers which are working at maximum capacity.

The Real Gonadotrophins

Two hormones known in the female as follicle stimulating hormone (FSH) and corpus luteum stimulating hormone (LSH) are secreted by the anterior lobe of the pituitary gland. These hormones are real gonadotrophins because they directly govern the function of the ovaries. The anterior pituitary is in turn governed by the diencephalon, and so when there is an ovarian deficiency the diencephalic center concerned is hard put to correct matters by increasing the secretion from the anterior pituitary of FSH or LSH, as the case may be. When sexual deficiency is clinically present, this is a sign that the diencephalic center concerned is unable, in spite of maximal exertion, to cope with the demand for anterior pituitary stimulation.[6] When then the administration of HCG increases the functional capacity of the diencephalon, all demands can be fully satisfied and the sex deficiency is corrected.

"...this is the true mechanism underlying the presumed gonadotrophic action of HCG is confirmed..."

That this is the true mechanism underlying the presumed gonadotrophic action of HCG is confirmed by the fact that when the pituitary gland of infantile rats is removed before they are given HCG, the latter has no effect on their sex-glands. HCG cannot therefore have a direct sex gland stimulating action like that of the anterior pituitary gonadotrophins, as FSH and LSH are justly called. The latter are entirely different substances from that which can be extracted from pregnancy urine and which, unfortunately, is called chorionic gonadotrophin. It would be no more clumsy, and certainly far more appropriate, if HCG were henceforth called chorionic diencephalotrophin.

Section Five: **Human Chorionic Gonadotropin (HCG)**

HCG no Sex Hormone

"...HCG is not a sex hormone..."

It cannot he sufficiently emphasized that HCG is not a sex-hormone, that its action is identical in men, women, children and in those cases in which the sex-glands no longer function owing to old age or their surgical removal. The only sexual change it can bring about after puberty is an improvement of a pre-existing deficiency, but never a stimulation beyond the normal. In an indirect way via the anterior pituitary, HCG regulates menstruation and facilitates conception, but it never virilizes a woman or feminizes a man. It neither makes men grow breasts nor does it interfere with their virility, though where this was deficient it may improve it. It never makes women grow a beard or develop a gruff voice. I have stressed this point only for the sake of my lay readers, because, it is our daily experience that when patients hear the word hormone they immediately jump to the conclusion that this must have something to do with the sex-sphere. They are not accustomed as we are, to think thyroid, insulin, cortisone, adrenalin etc, as hormones.

Importance and Potency of HCG

"...HCG has been known for over half a century."

Owing to the fact that HCG has no direct action on any endocrine gland, its enormous importance in pregnancy has been overlooked and its potency underestimated. Though a pregnant woman can produce as much as one million units per day, we find that the injection of only 125 units per day is ample to reduce weight at the rate of roughly one pound per day, even in a colossus weighing 400 pounds, when associated with a 500- Calorie diet. It is no exaggeration to say that the flooding of the female body with HCG is by far the most spectacular hormonal event in pregnancy. It has an enormous protective importance for mother and child, and I even go so far as to say that no woman, and certainly not an obese one, could carry her pregnancy to term without it.

"HCG has certainly been their Cinderella..."

If I can be forgiven for comparing my fellow-endocrinologists with wicked Godmothers, HCG has certainly been their Cinderella, and I can only romantically hope that its extraordinary effect on abnormal fat will prove to be its Fairy Godmother.

HCG has been known for over half a century. It is the substance which Aschheim and Zondek so brilliantly used to diagnose early pregnancy out of the urine. Apart from that, the only thing it did in the experimental laboratory was to produce precocious rats, and that was not particularly stimulating to further research at a time when much more thrilling endocrinological discoveries were pouring in from all sides, sweeping, HCG into the stiller back waters.

Section Five: **Obesity & Complicating Disorders**

"...complicating disorders are often associated with obesity, and these we must briefly discuss."

Some complicating disorders are often associated with obesity, and these we must briefly discuss. The most important associated disorders and the ones in which obesity seems to play a precipitating or at least an aggravating role are the following: the stable type of diabetes, gout, rheumatism and arthritis, high blood pressure and hardening of the arteries, coronary disease and cerebral hemorrhage.

Apart from the fact that they are often - though not necessarily - associated with obesity, these disorders have two things in common. In all of them, modern research is becoming more and more inclined to believe that diencephalic regulations play a dominant role in their causation. The other common factor is that they either improve or do not occur during pregnancy. In the latter respect they are joined by many other disorders not necessarily associated with obesity. Such disorders are, for instance, colitis, duodenal or gastric ulcers, certain allergies, psoriasis, loss of hair, brittle fingernails, migraine, etc.

If HCG + diet does in the obese bring about those diencephalic changes which are characteristic of pregnancy, one would expect to see an improvement in all these conditions comparable to that seen in real pregnancy. The administration of HCG does in fact do this in a remarkable way.

Diabetes

"...it is often possible to stop all antidiabetic medication after the first few days of treatment."

In an obese patient suffering from a fairly advanced case of stable diabetes of many years duration in which the blood sugar may range from 3-400 mg%, it is often possible to stop all antidiabetic medication after the first few days of treatment. The blood sugar continues to drop from day to day and often reaches normal values in 2-3 weeks. As in pregnancy, this phenomenon is not observed in the brittle type of diabetes, and as some cases that are predominantly stable may have a small brittle factor in their clinical makeup, all obese diabetics have to be kept under a very careful and expert watch.

A brittle case of diabetes is primarily due to the inability of the pancreas to produce sufficient insulin, while in the stable type, diencephalic regulations seem to be of greater importance. That is possibly the reason why the stable form responds so well to the HCG method of treating obesity, whereas the brittle type does not. Obese patients are generally suffering from the stable type, but a stable type may gradually change into a brittle one, which is usually associated with a loss of weight. Thus, when an obese diabetic finds that he is losing weight without diet or treatment, he should at once have his diabetes expertly attended to. There is some evidence to suggest that the change from stable to brittle is more liable to occur in patients who are taking insulin for their stable diabetes.

Rheumatism

"All rheumatic pains... improve subjectively within a few days of treatment..."

All rheumatic pains, even those associated with demonstrable bony lesions, improve subjectively within a few days of treatment, and often require neither cortisone nor salicylates. Again this is a well known phenomenon in pregnancy, and while under treatment with HCG + diet the effect is no less dramatic. As it does after pregnancy, the pain of deformed joints returns after treatment, but smaller doses of pain-relieving drugs seem able to control it satisfactorily after weight reduction. In any case, the HCG method makes it possible in obese arthritic patients to interrupt prolonged cor-

Section Five: **Obesity & Complicating Disorders**

tisone treatment without a recurrence of pain. This in itself is most welcome, but there is the added advantage that the treatment stimulates the secretion of ACTH in a physiological manner and that this regenerates the adrenal cortex, which is apt to suffer under prolonged cortisone treatment.

Cholesterol

"...the proportion of free to esterified cholesterol is reversed during the treatment of obesity with HCG + diet..."

The exact extent to which the blood cholesterol is involved in hardening of the arteries, high blood pressure and coronary disease is not as yet known, but it is now widely admitted that the blood cholesterol level is governed by diencephalic mechanisms. The behavior of circulating cholesterol is therefore of particular interest during the treatment of obesity with HCG. Cholesterol circulates in two forms, which we call free and esterified. Normally these fractions are present in a proportion of about 25% free to 75% esterified cholesterol, and it is the latter fraction which damages the walls of the arteries. In pregnancy this proportion is reversed and it may he taken for granted that arteriosclerosis never gets worse during pregnancy for this very reason.

To my knowledge, the only other condition in which the proportion of free to esterified cholesterol is reversed during the treatment of obesity with HCG + diet, when exactly the same phenomenon takes place. This seems an important indication of how closely a patient under HCG treatment resembles a pregnant woman in diencephalic behavior.

When the total amount of circulating cholesterol is normal before treatment, this absolute amount is neither significantly increased nor decreased. But when an obese patient with an abnormally high cholesterol and already showing signs of arteriosclerosis is treated with HCG, his blood pressure drops and his coronary circulation seems to improve, and yet his total blood cholesterol may soar to heights never before reached.

"...the increase is mostly in the form of the not dangerous free cholesterol..."

At first this greatly alarmed us. But then we saw that the patients came to no harm even if treatment was continued and we found in follow-up examinations undertaken some months after treatment that the cholesterol was much better than it had been before treatment. As the increase is mostly in the form of the not dangerous free cholesterol, we gradually came to welcome the phenomenon. Today we believe that the rise is entirely due to the liberation of recent cholesterol deposits that have not yet undergone calcification in the arterial wall and therefore highly beneficial.

Gout

"...worth remembering that the disease does not occur in women of childbearing age."

An identical behavior is found in the blood uric acid level of patients suffering from gout. Predictably such patients get an acute and often severe attack after the first few days of HCG treatment but then remain entirely free of pain, in spite of the fact that their blood uric acid often shows a marked increase which may persist for several months after treatment. Those patients who have regained their normal weight remain free of symptoms regardless of what they eat, while those that require a second course of treatment get another attack of gout as soon as the second course is initiated. We do not yet know what diencephalic mechanisms are involved in gout; possibly emotional factors play a role, and it is worth remembering that the disease does not occur in women of childbearing age. We now give 2 tablets daily of ZYLORIC to all patients who give a history of gout and have a high blood uric acid level. In this way we can completely avoid attacks during treatment.

Section Five: **Obesity & Complicating Disorders**

Blood Pressure

Patients who have brought themselves to the brink of malnutrition by exaggerated dieting, laxatives etc, often have an abnormally low blood pressure. In these cases the blood pressure rises to normal values at the beginning of treatment and then very gradually drops, as it always does in patients with a normal blood pressure. Normal values are always regained a few days after the treatment is over. Of this lowering of the blood pressure during treatment the patients are not aware. When the blood pressure is abnormally high, and provided there are no detectable renal lesions, the pressure drops, as it usually does in pregnancy. The drop is often very rapid, so rapid in fact that it sometimes is advisable to slow down the process with pressure sustaining medication until the circulation has had a few days time to adjust itself to the new situation. On the other hand, among the thousands of cases treated, we have never seen any untoward incident which could be attributed to the rather sudden drop in high blood pressure.

When a woman suffering from high blood pressure becomes pregnant her blood pressure very soon drops, but after her confinement it may gradually rise back to its former level. Similarly, a high blood pressure present before HCG treatment tends to rise again after the treatment is over, though this is not always the case. But the former high levels are rarely reached, and we have gathered the impression that such relapses respond better to orthodox drugs such as Reserpine than before treatment.

Peptic Ulcers

In our cases of obesity with gastric or duodenal ulcers we have noticed a surprising subjective improvement in spite of a diet which would generally be considered most inappropriate for an ulcer patient. Here, too, there is a similarity with pregnancy, in which peptic ulcers hardly ever occur. However we have seen two cases with a previous history of several hemorrhages in which a bleeding occurred within 2 weeks of the end of treatment.

Psoriasis, Fingernails, Hair, Varicose Ulcers

As in pregnancy, psoriasis greatly improves during treatment but may relapse when the treatment is over. Most patients spontaneously report a marked improvement in the condition of brittle fingernails. The loss of hair not infrequently associated with obesity is temporarily arrested, though in very rare cases an increased loss of hair has been reported. I remember a case in which a patient developed a patchy baldness - so called alopecia areata - after a severe emotional shock, just before she was about to start an HCG treatment. Our dermatologist diagnosed the case as a particularly severe one, predicting that all the hair would be lost. He counseled against the reducing treatment, but in view of my previous experience and as the patient was very anxious not to postpone reducing, I discussed the matter with the dermatologist and it was agreed that, having fully acquainted the patient with the situation, the treatment should be started. During the treatment, which lasted four weeks, the further development of the bald patches was almost, if not quite, arrested; however, within a week of having finished the course of HCG, all the remaining hair fell out as predicted by the dermatologist. The interesting point is that the treatment was able to postpone this result but not to prevent it. The patient has now grown a new shock of hair of which she is justly proud.

"...the pressure drops, as it usually does in pregnancy."

"...a surprising subjective improvement in spite of a diet..."

"...psoriasis greatly improves during treatment but may relapse when the treatment is over."

Section Five: **Obesity & Complicating Disorders**

In obese patients with large varicose ulcers we were surprised to find that these ulcers heal rapidly under treatment with HCG. We have since treated non obese patients suffering from varicose ulcers with daily injections of HCG on normal diet with equally good results.

The "Pregnant" Male Misconception

"...HCG in no way interferes with his sex.

When a male patient hears that he is about to be put into a condition which in some respects resembles pregnancy, he is usually shocked and horrified. The physician must therefore carefully explain that this does not mean that he will be feminized and that HCG in no way interferes with his sex. He must be made to understand that in the interest of the propagation of the species nature provides for a perfect functioning of the regulatory headquarters in the diencephalon during pregnancy and that we are merely using this natural safeguard as a means of correcting the diencephalic disorder which is responsible for his overweight.

Table I   Summary of Complicating Disorders & Effect of HCG.

"Amazingly most side effects are beneficial."

Condition	Result of HCG Adminstration
Diabetes	Blood sugar drops, often possible to stop medications.
Rheumatism	Pain lessens and overall improvement within days.
Cholesterol	Improved levels 'good vs bad' and highly beneficial.
Gout	Does not occur.
Blood Pressure	Normalizes and decreases after HCG usage.
Peptic Ulcers	Subjective improvements are possible.
Psoriasis	Greatly improves, temporarily, while under treatment.
'Pregnant' male	A complete misconception. No sexual side effects

"Apart from the fact that they are often - though not necessarily - associated with obesity, these disorders have two things in common. In all of them, modern research is becoming more and more inclined to believe that diencephalic regulations play a dominant role in their causation. The other common factor is that they either improve or do not occur during pregnancy."

Dr. Simeons

Section Five: **Technique & Advisory Warnings**

"...what follows is mainly for the treating physician and most certainly not a do-it-yourself primer."

I must warn the lay reader that what follows is mainly for the treating physician and most certainly **not a do-it-yourself** primer. Many of the expressions used mean something entirely different to a qualified doctor than that which their common use implies, and only a physician can correctly interpret the symptoms which may arise during treatment. Any patient who thinks he can reduce by taking a few "shots" and eating less is not only sure to be disappointed but may be heading for serious trouble. The benefit the patient can derive from reading this part of the book is a fuller realization of how very important it is for him to follow to the letter his physician's instructions.

In treating obesity with the HCG + diet method we are handling what is perhaps the most complex organ in the human body. The diencephalon's functional equilibrium is delicately poised, so that whatever happens in one part has repercussions in others.

"In treating obesity with the HCG + diet method we are handling what is perhaps the most complex organ in the human body."

In obesity this balance is out of kilter and can only be restored if the technique I am about to describe is followed implicitly. Even seemingly insignificant deviations, particularly those that at first sight seem to be an improvement, are very liable to produce most disappointing results and even annul the effect completely.

For instance, if the diet is increased from 500 to 600 or 700 Calories, the loss of weight is quite unsatisfactory. If the daily dose of HCG is raised to 200 or more units daily its action often appears to be reversed, possibly because larger doses evoke diencephalic counter-regulations. On the other hand, the diencephalon is an extremely robust organ in spite of its unbelievable intricacy. From an evolutionary point of view it is one of the oldest organs in our body and its evolutionary history dates back more than 500 million years.

This has tendered it extraordinarily adaptable to all natural exigencies, and that is one of the main reasons why the human species was able to evolve. What its evolution did not prepare it for were the conditions to which human culture and civilization now expose it.

Patient History Taking

"...diencephalon's functional equilibrium is delicately poised, so that whatever happens in one part has repercussions in others."

When a patient first presents himself for treatment, we take a general history and note the time when the first signs of overweight were observed. We try to establish the highest weight the patient has ever had in his life (obviously excluding pregnancy), when this was, and what measures have hitherto been taken in an effort to reduce.

It has been our experience that those patients who have been taking thyroid preparations for long periods have a slightly lower average loss of weight under treatment with HCG than those who have never taken thyroid. This is even so in those patients who have been taking thyroid because they had an abnormally low basal metabolic rate. In many of these cases the low BMR is not due to any intrinsic deficiency of the thyroid gland, but rather to a lack of diencephalic stimulation of the thyroid gland via the anterior pituitary lobe. We never allow thyroid to be taken during treatment, and yet a BMR which was very low before treatment is usually found to be normal after a week or two of HCG + diet. Needless to say, this does not apply to those cases in which a thyroid deficiency has been produced by the surgical removal of a part of an overactive gland. It is also most important to ascertain whether the patient has taken diuretics (water eliminating pills) as this also decreases the weight loss under the HCG regimen.

Section Five: **The Duration of Treatment**

Returning to our procedure, we next ask the patient a few questions to which he is held to reply simply with "yes" or "no". These questions are: Do you suffer from headaches? rheumatic pains? menstrual disorders? constipation? breathlessness or exertion? swollen ankles? Do you consider yourself greedy? Do you feel the need to eat snacks between meals?

"...normal weight for his height, age, skeletal and muscular build is established..."

The patient then strips and is weighed and measured. The normal weight for his height, age, skeletal and muscular build is established from tables of statistical averages, whereby in women it is often necessary to make an allowance for particularly large and heavy breasts. The degree of overweight is then calculated, and from this the duration of treatment can be roughly assessed on the basis of an average loss of weight of a little less than a pound, say 300-400 grams-per injection, per day. It is a particularly interesting feature of the HCG treatment that in reasonably cooperative patients this figure is remarkably constant, regardless of sex, age and degree of overweight.

The Duration of Treatment

Patients who need to lose 15 pounds (7 kg.) or less require 26 days treatment with 23 daily injections. The extra three days are needed because all patients must continue the 500-Calorie diet for three days after the last injection. This is a very essential part of the treatment, because if they start eating normally as long as there is even a trace of HCG in their body they put on weight alarmingly at the end of the treatment. After three days when all the HCG has been eliminated this does not happen, because the blood is then no longer saturated with food and can thus accommodate an extra influx from the intestines without increasing its volume by retaining water.

"...all patients must continue the 500-Calorie diet for three days..."

We never give a treatment lasting less than 26 days, even in patients needing to lose only 5 pounds. It seems that even in the mildest cases of obesity the diencephalon requires about three weeks rest from the maximal exertion to which it has been previously subjected in order to regain fully its normal fat-banking capacity. Clinically this expresses itself, in the fact that, when in these mild cases, treatment is stopped as soon as the weight is normal, which may be achieved in a week, it is much more easily regained than after a full course of 23 injections.

"...because HCG puts only abnormal fat into circulation..."

As soon as such patients have lost all their abnormal superfluous fat, they at once begin to feel ravenously hungry in spite of continued injections. This is because HCG puts only abnormal fat into circulation and cannot, in the doses used, liberate normal fat deposits; indeed, it seems to prevent their consumption. As soon as their statistically normal weight is reached, these patients are put on 800-1000 Calories for the rest of the treatment.

The diet is arranged in such a way that the weight remains perfectly stationary and is thus continued for three days after the 23rd injection. Only then are the patients free to eat anything they please except sugar and starches for the next three weeks.

Such early cases are common among actresses, models, and persons who are tired of obesity, having seen its ravages in other members of their family. Film actresses frequently explain that they must weigh less than normal. With this request we flatly refuse to comply, first, because we undertake to cure a disorder, not to create a new one, and second, because it is in the nature of the HCG method that it is self limiting. It be-

"...they see that under HCG their figure improves out of all proportion..."

comes completely ineffective as soon as all abnormal fat is consumed. Actresses with a slight tendency to obesity, having tried all manner of reducing methods, invariably come to the conclusion that their figure is satisfactory only when they are underweight, simply because none of these methods remove their superfluous fat deposits. When they see that under HCG their figure improves out of all proportion to the amount of weight lost, they are nearly always content to remain within their normal weight-range.

When a patient has more than 15 pounds to lose the treatment takes longer but the maximum we give in a single course is 40 injections, nor do we as a rule allow patients to lose more than 34 lbs. (15 Kg.) at a time. The treatment is stopped when either 34 lbs. have been lost or 40 injections have been given. The only exception we make is in the case of grotesquely obese patients who may be allowed to lose an additional 5-6 lbs. if this occurs before the 40 injections are up.

Immunity to HCG

The reason for limiting a course to 40 injections is that by then some patients may begin to show signs of HCG immunity. Though this phenomenon is well known, we cannot as yet define the underlying mechanism. Maybe after a certain length of time the body learns to break down and eliminate HCG very rapidly, or possibly prolonged treatment leads to some sort of counter-regulation which annuls the diencephalic effect.

After 40 daily injections it takes about six weeks before this so called immunity is lost and HCG again becomes fully effective. Usually after about 40 injections patients may feel the onset of immunity as hunger which was previously absent. In those comparatively rare cases in which signs of immunity develop before the full course of 40 injections has been completed-say at the 35th injection- treatment must be stopped at once, because if it is continued the patients begin to look weary and drawn, feel weak and hungry and any further loss of weight achieved is then always at the expense of normal fat. This is not only undesirable, but normal fat is also instantly regained as soon as the patient is returned to a free diet.

"...some patients may begin to show signs of HCG immunity."

Patients who need only 23 injections may be injected daily, including Sundays, as they never develop immunity. In those that take 40 injections the onset of immunity can be delayed if they are given only six injections a week, leaving out Sundays or any other day they choose, provided that it is always the same day. On the days on which they do not receive the injections they usually feel a slight sensation of hunger. At first we thought that this might be purely psychological, but we found that when normal saline is injected without the patient's knowledge the same phenomenon occurs.

Menstruation

"During menstruation no injections are given, but the diet is continued and causes no hardship..."

During menstruation no injections are given, but the diet is continued and causes no hardship; yet as soon as the menstruation is over, the patients become extremely hungry unless the injections are resumed at once. It is very impressive to see the suffering of a woman who has continued her diet for a day or two beyond the end of the period without coming for her injection and then to hear the next day that all hunger ceased within a few hours after the injection and to see her once again content, florid and cheerful. While on the question of menstruation it must he added that in teenaged girls the period may in some rare cases be delayed and exceptionally stop altogether. If then later this is artificially induced some weight may be regained.

Further Courses

"Patients requiring the loss of more than 34 lbs. must have a second or even more courses."

Patients requiring the loss of more than 34 lbs. must have a second or even more courses. A second course can be started after an interval of not less than six weeks, though the pause can be more than six weeks. When a third, fourth or even fifth course is necessary, the interval between courses should be made progressively longer. Between a second and third course eight weeks should elapse, between a third and fourth course twelve weeks, between a fourth and fifth course twenty weeks and between a fifth and sixth course six months. In this way it is possible to bring about a weight reduction of 100 lbs. and more if required without the least hardship to the patient.

In general, men do slightly better than women and often reach a somewhat higher average daily loss. Very advanced cases do a little better than early ones, but it is a remarkable fact that this difference is only just statistically significant.

"In general, men do slightly better than women..."

Conditions That Must Be Accepted Before Treatment

On the basis of these data the probable duration of treatment can he calculated with considerable accuracy, and this is explained to the patient. It is made clear to him that during the course of treatment he must attend the clinic daily to be weighed, injected and generally checked. All patients that live in Rome or have resident friends or relations with whom they can stay are treated as out-patients, but patients coming from abroad must stay in the hospital, as no hotel or restaurant can be relied upon to prepare the diet with sufficient accuracy. These patients have their meals, sleep, and attend the clinic in the hospital, but are otherwise free to spend their time as they please in the city and its surroundings sightseeing, bathing or theater-going.

"...a patient can only consider himself really cured when he has been reduced to his statistically normal weight..."

It is also made clear that between courses the patient gets no treatment and is free to eat anything he pleases except starches and sugar during the first 3 weeks. It is impressed upon him that he will have to follow the prescribed diet to the letter and that after the first three days this will cost him no effort, as he will feel no hunger and may indeed have difficulty in getting down the 500 Calories which he will be given. If these conditions are not acceptable the case is refused, as any compromise or half measure is bound to prove utterly disappointing to patient and physician alike and is a waste of time and energy.

Though a patient can only consider himself really cured when he has been reduced to his statistically normal weight, we do not insist that he commit himself to that extent. Even a partial loss of overweight is highly beneficial, and it is our experience that once a patient has completed a first course he is so enthusiastic about the ease with which the - to him surprising - results are achieved that he almost invariably comes back for more. There certainly can be no doubt that in my clinic more time is spent on damping over-enthusiasm than on insisting that the rules of the treatment be observed.

Section Five: **Examining the Patient**

"One cannot keep a patient comfortably on 500 Calories unless his normal fat reserves are reasonably well stocked."

Only when agreement is reached on the points so far discussed do we proceed with the examination of the patient. A note is made of the size of the first upper incisor, of a pad of fat on the nape of the neck, at the axilla and on the inside of the knees. The presence of striation, a suprapubic fold, a thoracic fold, angulation of elbow and knee joint, breast-development in men and women, edema of the ankles and the state of genital development in the male are noted.

Wherever this seems indicated we X-ray the sella turcica, as the bony capsule which contains the pituitary gland is called, measure the basal metabolic rate, X-ray the chest and take an electrocardiogram. We do a blood-count and a sedimentation rate and estimate uric acid, cholesterol, iodine and sugar in the fasting blood.

Gain before Loss

Patients whose general condition is low, owing to excessive previous dieting, must eat to capacity for about one week before starting treatment, regardless of how much weight they may gain in the process. One cannot keep a patient comfortably on 500 Calories unless his normal fat reserves are reasonably well stocked. It is for this reason also that every case, even those that are actually gaining must eat to capacity of the most fattening food they can get down until they have had the third injection. It is a fundamental mistake to put a patient on 500 Calories as soon as the injections are started, as it seems to take about three injections before abnormally deposited fat begins to circulate and thus become available.

We distinguish between the first three injections, which we call "non-effective" as far as the loss of weight is concerned, and the subsequent injections given while the patient is dieting, which we call "effective". The average loss of weight is calculated on the number of effective injections and from the weight reached on the day of the third injection which may be well above what it was two days earlier when the first injection was given.

"...are very hard to convince of the absolute necessity of gorging for at least two days..."

Most patients who have been struggling with diets for years and know how rapidly they gain if they let themselves go are very hard to convince of the absolute necessity of gorging for at least two days, and yet this must he insisted upon categorically if the further course of treatment is to run smoothly. Those patients who have to be put on forced feeding for a week before starting the injections usually gain weight rapidly - four to six pounds in 24 hours is not unusual - but after a day or two this rapid gain generally levels off. In any case, the whole gain is usually lost in the first 48 hours of dieting. It is necessary to proceed in this manner because the gain re-stocks the depleted normal reserves, whereas the subsequent loss is from the abnormal deposits only.

Patients in a satisfactory general condition and those who have not just previously restricted their diet start forced feeding on the day of the first injection. Some patents say that they can no longer overeat because their stomach has shrunk after years of restrictions. While we know that no stomach ever shrinks, we compromise by insisting that they eat frequently of highly concentrated foods such as milk chocolate, pastries with whipped cream sugar, fried meats (particularly pork), eggs and bacon, mayonnaise, bread with thick butter and jam, etc. The time and trouble spent on pressing this point upon incredulous or reluctant patients is always amply rewarded afterwards by the complete absence of those difficulties which patients who have disregarded these instructions are liable to experience.

Section Five: **Starting Treatment**

During the two days of forced feeding from the first to the third injection - many patients are surprised that contrary to their previous experience they do not gain weight and some even lose. The explanation is that in these cases there is a compensatory flow of urine, which drains excessive water from the body. To some extent this seems to be a direct action of HCG, but it may also be due to a higher protein intake, as we know that a protein-deficient diet makes the body retain water.

"...many patients are surprised that contrary to their previous experience they do not gain weight..."

Starting treatment

In menstruating women, the best time to start treatment is immediately after a period. Treatment may also be started later, but it is advisable to have at least ten days in hand before the onset of the next period. Similarly, the end of a course of HCG should never be made to coincide with menstruation. If things should happen to work out that way, it is better to give the last injection three days before the expected date of the menses so that a normal diet can he resumed at onset. Alternatively, at least three injections should be given after the period, followed by the usual three days of dieting. This rule need not be observed in such patients who have reached their normal weight before the end of treatment and are already on a higher caloric diet.

"...but it may also be due to a higher protein intake..."

Patients who require more than the minimum of 23 injections and who therefore skip one day a week in order to postpone immunity to HCG cannot have their third injections on the day before the interval. Thus if it is decided to skip Sundays, the treatment can be started on any day of the week except Thursdays. Supposing they start on Thursday, they will have their third injection on Saturday, which is also the day on which they start their 500 Calorie diet. They would then have no injection on the second day of dieting; this exposes them to an unnecessary hardship, as without the injection they will feel particularly hungry. Of course, the difficulty can be overcome by exceptionally injecting them on the first Sunday. If this day falls between the first and second or between the second and third injection, we usually prefer to give the patient the extra day of forced feeding, which the majority rapturously enjoy.

Table J   Starting HCG Treatment - First Course 'Gorge Days"

Here's What the Doctor is Talking about. 'Pig Out' required!

"...to clarify the proper use of the 'gorge days.'

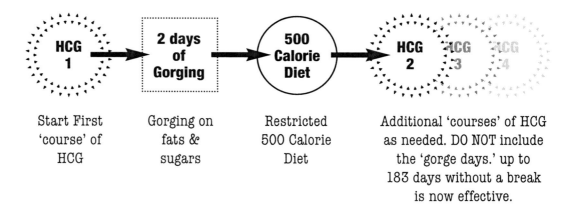

Start First 'course' of HCG | Gorging on fats & sugars | Restricted 500 Calorie Diet | Additional 'courses' of HCG as needed. DO NOT include the 'gorge days.' up to 183 days without a break is now effective.

Section Five: **The 500 Calorie Diet**

The 500 Calorie diet is explained on the day of the second injection to those patients who will be preparing their own food, and it is most important that the person who will actually cook is present - the wife, the mother or the cook, as the case may be. Here in Italy patients are given the following diet sheet.

Breakfast:

Tea or coffee in any quantity without sugar. Only one tablespoonful of milk allowed in 24 hours. Saccharin or Stevia may be used.

"... it is most important that the person who will actually cook is present - the wife, the mother or the cook..."

Lunch:

Protein: 100 grams of veal, beef, chicken breast, fresh white fish, lobster, crab, or shrimp. All visible fat must be carefully removed before cooking, and the meat must be weighed raw. It must be boiled or grilled without additional fat. Salmon, eel, tuna, herring, dried or pickled fish are not allowed. The chicken breast must be removed from the bird.

Vegetable: One type of vegetable only to be chosen from the following: spinach, chard, chicory, beet-greens, green salad, tomatoes, celery, fennel, onions, red radishes, cucumbers, asparagus, cabbage.

Breads: One breadstick (grissino) or one Melba toast.

Fruit: An apple, orange, or one-half grapefruit.

Dinner:

Choose from the same four groups as lunch shown above BUT avoid the same choice twice in a row. i.e. if you have chicken for lunch then have a **different protein** choice for dinner.

Condiments & Seasonings:

The juice of **one lemon daily** is allowed for all purposes. Salt, pepper, vinegar, mustard powder, garlic, sweet basil, parsley, thyme, majoram, etc., if they contain **NO SUGAR**, may be used for seasoning. **NO OIL**, butter or dressing.

Drinks & Fluid Intake:

"...the patient should drink about 2 liters of these fluids per day..."

Tea, coffee, plain water, or mineral water are the only drinks allowed, but they may be taken in any quantity and at all times. Remember **NO SUGAR**.

In fact, the patient should drink about **2 liters** of these fluids **per day**. Many patients are afraid to drink so much because they fear that this may make them retain more water. This is a wrong notion as the body is more inclined to store water when the intake falls below its normal requirements.

The fruit or the breadstick may be eaten between meals instead of at lunch or dinner, but not more than than four items, one in each category listed, may be eaten at one meal. Remember to alternate your choices.

No medicines or cosmetics other than lipstick, eyebrow pencil and powder may be used without special permission.

Every item in the list is gone over carefully, continually stressing the point that no variations other than those listed may be introduced. All things not listed are forbidden, and the patient is assured that nothing permissible has been left out. The 100 grams of meat must he scrupulously weighed raw after all visible fat has been removed. To do this accurately the patient must have a letter-scale, as kitchen scales are not sufficiently accurate and the butcher should certainly not be relied upon. Those not uncommon patients who feel that even so little food is too much for them, can omit anything they wish.

"No medicines or cosmetics other than lipstick, eyebrow pencil and powder may be used without special permission."

There is no objection to breaking up the two meals. For instance having a breadstick and an apple for breakfast or an orange before going to bed, provided they are deducted from the regular meals. The whole daily ration of two breadsticks or two fruits may not be eaten at the same time, nor can any item saved from the previous day be added on the following day. In the beginning patients are advised to check every meal against their diet sheet before starting to eat and not to rely on their memory. It is also worth pointing out that any attempt to observe this diet without HCG will lead to trouble in two to three days. We have had cases in which patients have proudly flaunted their dieting powers in front of their friends without mentioning the fact that they are also receiving treatment with HCG. They let their friends try the same diet, and when this proves to be a failure - as it necessarily must - the patient starts raking in unmerited kudos for superhuman willpower.

"There is no objection to breaking up the two meals."

It should also be mentioned that two small apples weighing as much as one large one never the less have a higher caloric value and are therefore not allowed though there is no restriction on the size of one apple. Some people do not realize that a tangerine is not an orange and that chicken breast does not mean the breast of any other fowl, nor does it mean a wing or drumstick.

The most tiresome patients are those who start counting Calories and then come up with all manner of ingenious variations which they compile from their little books. When one has spent years of weary research trying to make a diet as attractive as possible without jeopardizing the loss of weight, culinary geniuses who are out to improve their unhappy lot are hard to take.

"...culinary geniuses who are out to improve their unhappy lot are hard to take."

Making up the Calories on the HCG 500 Calorie Diet

The diet used in conjunction with HCG must not exceed 500 Calories per day, and the way these Calories are made up is of utmost importance. For instance, if a patient drops the apple and eats an extra breadstick instead, he will not be getting more Calories but he will not lose weight. There are a number of foods, particularly fruits and vegetables, which have the same or even lower caloric values than those listed as permissible, and yet we find that they interfere with the regular loss of weight under HCG, presumably owing to the nature of their composition. Pimiento peppers, okra, artichokes and pears are examples of this.

While this diet works satisfactorily in Italy, certain modifications have to be made in other countries. For instance, American beef has almost double the caloric value of South Italian beef, which is not marbled with fat. This marbling is impossible to re-

Section Five: **Precautions & Guidelines**

"...it must be borne in mind that the total daily intake must not exceed 500 Calories..."

move. In America, therefore, low-grade veal should be used for one meal and fish (excluding all those species such as herring, mackerel, tuna, salmon, eel, etc., which have a high fat content, and all dried, smoked or pickled fish), chicken breast, lobster, crawfish, prawns, shrimps, crabmeat or kidneys for the other meal. Where the Italian breadsticks, the so-called grissini, are not available, one Melba toast may be used instead, though they are psychologically less satisfying. A Melba toast has about the same weight as the very porous grissini which is much more to look at and to chew.

In many countries specially prepared unsweetened and low Calorie foods are freely available, and some of these can be tentatively used. When local conditions or the feeding habits of the population make changes necessary it must be borne in mind that the total daily intake must not exceed 500 Calories if the best possible results are to be obtained, that the daily ration should contain 200 grams of fat-free protein and a very small amount of starch.

Just as the daily dose of HCG is the same in all cases, so the same diet proves to be satisfactory for a small elderly lady of leisure or a hard working muscular giant. Under the effect of HCG the obese body is always able to obtain all the Calories it needs from the abnormal fat deposits, regardless of whether it uses up 1500 or 4000 per day. It must be made very clear to the patient that he is living to a far greater extent on the fat which he is losing than on what he eats.

"Under the effect of HCG the obese body is always able to obtain all the Calories it needs..."

Many patients ask why eggs are not allowed. The contents of two good sized eggs are roughly equivalent to 100 grams of meat, but unfortunately the yolk contains a large amount of fat, which is undesirable. Very occasionally we allow egg - boiled, poached or raw - to patients who develop an aversion to meat, but in this case they must add the white of three eggs to the one they eat whole. In countries where cottage cheese made from skimmed milk is available 100 grams may occasionally be used instead of the meat, but no other cheeses are allowed.

Vegetarians

Strict vegetarians such as orthodox Hindus present a special problem, because milk and curds are the only animal protein they will eat. To supply them with sufficient protein of animal origin they must drink 500 cc. of skimmed milk per day, though part of this ration can be taken as curds. As far as fruit, vegetables and starch are concerned, their diet is the same as that of non-vegetarians; they cannot be allowed their usual intake of vegetable proteins from leguminous plants such as beans or from wheat or nuts, nor can they have their customary rice. In spite of these severe restrictions, their average loss is about half that of non-vegetarians, presumably owing to the sugar content of the milk.

"...the slightest deviation from the diet has under HCG disastrous results as far as the weight is concerned..."

Faulty Dieting

Few patients will take one's word for it that the slightest deviation from the diet has under HCG disastrous results as far as the weight is concerned. This extreme sensitivity has the advantage that the smallest error is immediately detectable at the daily weighing but most patients have to make the experience before they will believe it.

Persons in high official positions such as embassy personnel, politicians, senior executives, etc., who are obliged to attend social functions to which they cannot bring

"...only the actual fat is burned up; all the vitamins, the proteins, the blood, and the minerals which this tissue contains in abundance are fed back into the body."

their meager meal must be told beforehand that an official dinner will cost them the loss of about three days treatment, however careful they are and in spite of a friendly and would-be cooperative host. We generally advise them to avoid all-round embarrassment, the almost inevitable turn of conversation to their weight problem and the outpouring of lay counsel from their table partners by not letting it be known that they are under treatment. They should take dainty servings of everything, hide what they can under the cutlery and book the gain which may take three days to get rid of as one of the sacrifices which their profession entails. Allowing three days for their correction, such incidents do not jeopardize the treatment, provided they do not occur all too frequently in which case treatment should be postponed to a socially more peaceful season.

Vitamins and Anemia

Sooner or later most patients express a fear that they may be running out of vitamins or that the restricted diet may make them anemic. On this score the physician can confidently relieve their apprehension by explaining that every time they lose a pound of fatty tissue, which they do almost daily, only the actual fat is burned up; all the vitamins, the proteins, the blood, and the minerals which this tissue contains in abundance are fed back into the body. Actually, a low blood count not due to any serious disorder of the blood forming tissues improves during treatment, and we have never encountered a significant protein deficiency nor signs of a lack of vitamins in patients who are dieting regularly.

The First Days of Treatment

"...I am longing to get on with your diet."

On the day of the third injection it is almost routine to hear two remarks. One is: "You know, Doctor, I'm sure it's only psychological, but I already feel quite different". So common is this remark, even from very skeptical patients that we hesitate to accept the psychological interpretation. The other typical remark is: "Now that I have been allowed to eat anything I want, I can't get it down. Since yesterday I feel like a stuffed pig. Food just doesn't seem to interest me any more, and I am longing to get on with your diet". Many patients notice that they are passing more urine and that the swelling in their ankles is less even before they start dieting.

On the day of the fourth injection most patients declare that they are feeling fine. They have usually lost two pounds or more, some say they feel a bit empty but hasten to explain that this does not amount to hunger. Some complain of a mild headache of which they have been forewarned and for which they have been given permission to take aspirin.

"...a difference appears between those patients who have literally eaten to capacity during the first two days of treatment..."

During the second and third day of dieting - that is, the fifth and sixth injection-these minor complaints improve while the weight continues to drop at about double the usually overall average of almost one pound per day, so that a moderately severe case may by the fourth day of dieting have lost as much as 8- 10 lbs.

It is usually at this point that a difference appears between those patients who have literally eaten to capacity during the first two days of treatment and those who have not. The former feel remarkably well; they have no hunger, nor do they feel tempted when others eat normally at the same table. They feel lighter, more clear-headed and notice a desire to move quite contrary to their previous lethargy. Those who have dis-

Section Five: **Precautions & Guidelines**

regarded the advice to eat to capacity continue to have minor discomforts and do not have the same euphoric sense of well-being until about a week later. It seems that their normal fat reserves require that much more time before they are fully stocked.

Fluctuations in weight loss

"...women are more irregular in spite of faultless dieting."

After the fourth or fifth day of dieting the daily loss of weight begins to decrease to one pound or somewhat less per day, and there is a smaller urinary output. Men often continue to lose regularly at that rate, but women are more irregular in spite of faultless dieting. There may be no drop at all for two or three days and then a sudden loss which reestablishes the normal average. These fluctuations are entirely due to variations in the retention and elimination of water, which are more marked in women than in men.

"Under the influence of HCG, fat is being extracted from the cells, in which it is stored in the fatty tissue."

The weight registered by the scale is determined by two processes not necessarily synchronized. Under the influence of HCG, fat is being extracted from the cells, in which it is stored in the fatty tissue. When these cells are empty and therefore serve no purpose, the body breaks down the cellular structure and absorbs it, but breaking up of useless cells, connective tissue, blood vessels, etc., may lag behind the process of fat-extraction. When this happens the body appears to replace some of the extracted fat with water which is retained for this purpose. As water is heavier than fat the scales may show no loss of weight, although sufficient fat has actually been consumed to make up for the deficit in the 500-Calorie diet. When then such tissue is finally broken down, the water is liberated and there is a sudden flood of urine and a marked loss of weight. This simple interpretation of what is really an extremely complex mechanism is the one we give those patients who want to know why it is that on certain days they do not lose, though they have committed no dietary error.

"Diuretics should never be used for reducing."

Patients who have previously regularly used diuretics as a method of reducing, lose fat during the first two or three weeks of treatment which shows in their measurements, but the scale may show little or no loss because they are replacing the normal water content of their body which has been dehydrated. Diuretics should never be used for reducing.

Section Five: **Four Interruptions of Weight Loss**

We distinguish **four types of interruption** in the regular daily loss.

ONE: Stationary

"...the weight stays stationary for a day or two..."

The first is the one that has already been mentioned in which the weight stays stationary for a day or two, and this occurs, particularly towards the end of a course, in almost every case.

TWO: The Plateau

The second type of interruption we call a "plateau". A plateau lasts 4-6 days and frequently occurs during the second half of a full course, particularly in patients that have been doing well and whose overall average of nearly a pound per effective injection has been maintained. Those who are losing more than the average all have a plateau sooner or later. A plateau always corrects, itself, but many patients who have become accustomed to a regular daily loss get unnecessarily worried and begin to fret. No amount of explanation convinces them that a plateau does not mean that they are no longer responding normally to treatment.

"A plateau lasts 4-6 days and frequently occurs during the second half of a full course..."

In such cases we consider it permissible, for purely psychological reasons, to break up the plateau. This can be done in two ways. One is a so-called "apple day". An apple-day begins at lunch and continues until just before lunch of the following day. The patients are given six large apples and are told to eat one whenever they feel the desire though six apples is the maximum allowed. During an apple-day no other food or liquids except plain water are allowed and of water they may only drink just enough to quench an uncomfortable thirst if eating an apple still leaves them thirsty. Most patients feel no need for water and are quite happy with their six apples. Needless to say, an apple-day may never be given on the day on which there is no injection. The apple-day produces a gratifying loss of weight on the following day, chiefly due to the elimination of water. This water is not regained when the patients resume their normal 500-Calorie diet at lunch, and on the following days they continue to lose weight satisfactorily.

"This can be done in two ways. One is a so-called "apple day.""

The other way to break up a plateau is by giving a non-mercurial diuretic **[7]** for one day. This is simpler for the patient but we prefer the apple-day as we sometimes find that though the diuretic is very effective on the following day it may take two to three days before the normal daily reduction is resumed, throwing the patient into a new fit of despair. It is useless to give either an apple-day or a diuretic unless the weight has been stationary for at least four days without any dietary error having been committed.

THREE: Reaching a Former Level

The third type of interruption in the regular loss of weight may last much longer - ten days to two weeks. Fortunately, it is rare and only occurs in very advanced cases, and then hardly ever during the first course of treatment. It is seen only in those patients who during some period of their lives have maintained a certain fixed degree of obesity for ten years or more and have then at some time rapidly increased beyond that weight. When then in the course of treatment the former level is reached, it may take two weeks of no loss, in spite of HCG and diet, before further reduction is normally resumed.

FOUR: Menstrual Interruption

"...interruption of the normal loss of weight which does not fit perfectly into one of those categories is always due to some possibly very minor dietary error."

The fourth type of interruption is the one which often occurs a few days before and during the menstrual period and in some women at the time of ovulation. It must also be mentioned that when a woman becomes pregnant during treatment - and this is by no means uncommon - she at once ceases to lose weight. An unexplained arrest of reduction has on several occasions raised our suspicion before the first period was missed. If in such cases, menstruation is delayed, we stop injecting and do a precipitation test five days later. No pregnancy test should be carried out earlier than five days after the last injection, as otherwise the HCG may give a false positive result. Oral contraceptives may be used during treatment.

Dietary Errors

Any interruption of the normal loss of weight which does not fit perfectly into one of those categories is always due to some possibly very minor dietary error. Similarly, any gain of more than 100 grams is invariably the result of some transgression or mistake, unless it happens on or about the day of ovulation or during the three days preceding the onset of menstruation, in which case it is ignored. In all other cases the reason for the gain must be established at once.

"The patient who frankly admits that he has stepped out of his regimen when told that something has gone wrong is no problem."

The patient who frankly admits that he has stepped out of his regimen when told that something has gone wrong is no problem. He is always surprised at being found out, because unless he has seen this himself he will not believe that a salted almond, a couple of potato chips, a glass of tomato juice or an extra orange will bring about a definite increase in his weight on the following day.

Very often he wants to know why extra food weighing one ounce should increase his weight by six ounces. We explain this in the following way: Under the influence of HCG the blood is saturated with food and the blood volume has adapted itself so that it can only just accommodate the 500 Calories which come in from the intestinal tract in the course of the day. Any additional income, however little this may be, cannot be accommodated and the blood is therefore forced to increase its volume sufficiently to hold the extra food, which it can only do in a very diluted form. Thus it is not the weight of what is eaten that plays the determining role but rather the amount of water which the body must retain to accommodate this food.

This can be illustrated by mentioning the case of salt. In order to hold one teaspoonful of salt the body requires one liter of water, as it cannot accommodate salt in any higher concentration. Thus, if a person eats one teaspoonfull of salt his weight will go up by more than two pounds as soon as this salt is absorbed from his intestine.

"It must therefore be made clear that this only happens as long as they are under HCG."

To this explanation many patients reply: Well, if I put on that much every time I eat a little extra, how can I hold my weight after the treatment? It must therefore be made clear that this only happens as long as they are under HCG. When treatment is over, the blood is no longer saturated and can easily accommodate extra food without having to increase its volume. Here again the professional reader will be aware that this interpretation is a simplification of an extremely intricate physiological process which actually accounts for the phenomenon.

Section Five: **Dietary Errors & Other Factors**

Salt and Reducing

"...not in the least interested in such illusory weight losses as can be achieved by depriving the body of salt and by desiccating it."

While we are on the subject of salt, I can take this opportunity to explain that we make no restriction in the use of salt and insist that the patients drink large quantities of water throughout the treatment. We are out to reduce abnormal fat and are not in the least interested in such illusory weight losses as can be achieved by depriving the body of salt and by desiccating it. Though we allow the free use of salt, the daily amount taken should be roughly the same, as a sudden increase will of course be followed by a corresponding increase in weight as shown by the scale. An increase in the intake of salt is one of the most common causes for an increase in weight from one day to the next. Such an increase can be ignored, provided it is accounted for. It in no way influences the regular loss of fat.

Water

"...the amount of water they retain has nothing to do with the amount of water they drink."

Patients are usually hard to convince that the amount of water they retain has nothing to do with the amount of water they drink. When the body is forced to retain water, it will do this at all costs. If the fluid intake is insufficient to provide all the water required, the body withholds water from the kidneys and the urine becomes scanty and highly concentrated, imposing a certain strain on the kidneys. If that is insufficient, excessive water will be with-drawn from the intestinal tract, with the result that the feces become hard and dry. On the other hand if a patient drinks more than his body requires, the surplus is promptly and easily eliminated. Trying to prevent the body from retaining water by drinking less is not only futile but even harmful.

Constipation

"Once the patient realizes that it is in his own interest that he play an active and not merely a passive role in this search, the reason for the setback is almost invariably discovered."

An excess of water keeps the feces soft, and that is very important in the obese, who commonly suffer from constipation and a spastic colon. While a patient is under treatment we never permit the use of any kind of laxative taken by mouth. We explain that owing to the restricted diet it is perfectly satisfactory and normal to have an evacuation of the bowel only once every three to four days and that, provided plenty of fluids are taken, this never leads to any disturbance. Only in those patients who begin to fret after four days do we allow the use of a suppository. Patients who observe this rule find that after treatment they have a perfectly normal bowel action and this delights many of them almost as much as their loss of weight.

Investigating Dietary Errors

When the reason for a slight gain in weight is not immediately evident, it is necessary to investigate further. A patient who is unaware of having committed an error or is unwilling to admit a mistake protests indignantly when told he has done something he ought not to have done. In that atmosphere no fruitful investigation can be conducted; so we calmly explain that we are not accusing him of anything but that we know for certain from our not inconsiderable experience that something has gone wrong and that we must now sit down quietly together and try and find out what it was. Once the patient realizes that it is in his own interest that he play an active and not merely a passive role in this search, the reason for the setback is almost invariably discovered. Having been through hundreds of such sessions, we are nearly always able to distinguish the deliberate liar from the patient who is merely fooling himself or is really unaware of having erred.

Section Five: **Dietary Errors & Other Factors**

"...warn him that unless he comes clean we may refuse further treatment."

Liars and Fools

When we see obese patients there are generally two of us present in order to speed up routine handling. Thus when we have to investigate a rise in weight, a glance is sufficient to make sure that we agree or disagree. If after a few questions we both feel reasonably sure that the patient is deliberately lying, we tell him that this is our opinion and warn him that unless he comes clean we may refuse further treatment. The way he reacts to this furnishes additional proof whether we are on the right track or not we now very rarely make a mistake.

If the patient breaks down and confesses, we melt and are all forgiveness and treatment proceeds. Yet if such performances have to be repeated more than two or three times, we refuse further treatment. This happens in less than 1% of our cases. If the patient is stubborn and will not admit what he has been up to, we usually give him one more chance and continue treatment even though we have been unable to find the reason for his gain. In many such cases there is no repetition, and frequently the patient does then confess a few days later after he has thought things over.

"The patient who is fooling himself is the one who has committed some trifling, offense against the rules..."

The patient who is fooling himself is the one who has committed some trifling, offense against the rules but who has been able to convince himself that this is of no importance and cannot possibly account for the gain in weight. Women seem particularly prone to getting themselves entangled in such delusions. On the other hand, it does frequently happen that a patient will in the midst of a conversation unthinkingly spear an olive or forget that he has already eaten his breadstick.

A mother preparing food for the family may out of sheer habit forget that she must not taste the sauce to see whether it needs more salt. Sometimes a rich maiden aunt cannot be offended by refusing a cup of tea into which she has put two teaspoons of sugar, thoughtfully remembering the patient's taste from previous occasions. Such incidents are legion and are usually confessed without hesitation, but some patients seem genuinely able to forget these lapses and remember them with a visible shock only after insistent questioning.

In these cases we go carefully over the day. Sometimes the patient has been invited to a meal or gone to a restaurant, naively believing that the food has actually been prepared exactly according to instructions. They will say: "Yes, now that I come to think of it the steak did seem a bit bigger than the one I have at home, and it did taste better; maybe there was a little fat on it, though I specially told them to cut it all away". Sometimes the breadsticks were broken and a few fragments eaten, and "Maybe they were a little more than one". It is not uncommon for patients to place too much reliance on their memory of the diet-sheet and start eating carrots, beans or peas and then to seem genuinely surprised when their attention is called to the fact that these are forbidden, as they have not been listed.

"...fats, oils, creams and ointments applied to the skin are absorbed and interfere with weight reduction by HCG just as if they had been eaten."

Cosmetics

When no dietary error is elicited we turn to cosmetics. Most women find it hard to believe that fats, oils, creams and ointments applied to the skin are absorbed and interfere with weight reduction by HCG just as if they had been eaten. This almost incredible sensitivity to even such very minor increases in nutritional intake is a peculiar feature of the HCG method. For instance, we find that persons who

Section Five: **Dietary Errors & Other Factors**

"Under treatment normal fat is restored to the skin, which rapidly becomes fresh and turgid, making the expression much more youthful."

habitually handle organic fats, such as workers in beauty parlors, masseurs, butchers, etc. never show what we consider a satisfactory loss of weight unless they can avoid fat coming into contact with their skin.

The point is so important that I will illustrate it with two cases. A lady who was cooperating perfectly suddenly increased half a pound. Careful questioning brought nothing to light. She had certainly made no dietary error nor had she used any kind of face cream, and she was already in the menopause. As we felt that we could trust her implicitly, we left the question suspended. Yet just as she was about to leave the consulting room she suddenly stopped, turned and snapped her fingers. "I've got it," she said. This is what had happened : She had bought herself a new set of make-up pots and bottles and, using her fingers, had transferred her large assortment of cosmetics to the new containers in anticipation of the day she would be able to use them again after her treatment.

The other case concerns a man who impressed us as being very conscientious. He was about 20 lbs. overweight but did not lose satisfactorily from the onset of treatment. Again and again we tried to find the reason but with no success, until one day he said:"I never told you this, but I have a glass eye. In fact, I have a whole set of them. I frequently change them, and every time I do that I put a special ointment in my eye-socket.. Do you think that could have anything to do with it?" As we thought just that, we asked him to stop using this ointment, and from that day on his weight-loss was regular.

"...another interesting feature of the HCG method is that it does not ruin a singing voice."

We are particularly averse to those modern cosmetics which contain hormones, as any interference with endocrine regulations during treatment must be absolutely avoided. Many women whose skin has in the course of years become adjusted to the use of fat containing cosmetics find that their skin gets dry as soon as they stop using them. In such cases we permit the use of plain mineral oil, which has no nutritional value. On the other hand, mineral oil should not be used in preparing the food, first because of its undesirable laxative quality, and second because it absorbs some fat-soluble vitamins, which are then lost in the stool. We do permit the use of lipstick, powder and such lotions as are entirely free of fatty substances. We also allow brilliantine to be used on the hair but it must not be rubbed into the scalp. Obviously suntan oil is prohibited.

Many women are horrified when told that for the duration of treatment they cannot use face creams or have facial massages. They fear that this and the loss of weight will ruin their complexion. They can be fully reassured. Under treatment normal fat is restored to the skin, which rapidly becomes fresh and turgid, making the expression much more youthful. This is a characteristic of the HCG method which is a constant source of wonder to patients who have experienced or seen in others the facial ravages produced by the usual methods of reducing. An obese woman of 70 obviously cannot expect to have her pued face reduced to normal without a wrinkle, but it is remarkable how youthful her face remains in spite of her age.

The Voice is Not Affected by HCG

Incidentally, another interesting feature of the HCG method is that it does not ruin a singing voice. The typically obese prima donna usually finds that when she tries to reduce, the timbre of her voice is liable to change, and understandably this terrifies her. Under HCG this does not happen; indeed, in many cases the voice improves and the breathing invariably does. We have had many cases of professional singers very carefully controlled by expert voice teachers, and the maestros have been so enthusiastic that they now frequently send us patients.

Other Reasons for a Gain

"Apart from diet and cosmetics there can be a few other reasons for a small rise in weight."

Apart from diet and cosmetics there can be a few other reasons for a small rise in weight. Some patients unwittingly take chewing gum, throat pastilles, vitamin pills, cough syrups etc., without realizing that the sugar or fats they contain may interfere with a regular loss of weight. Sex hormones or cortisone in its various modern forms must be avoided, though oral contraceptives are permitted. In fact the only self-medication we allow is aspirin for a headache, though headaches almost invariably disappear after a week of treatment, particularly if of the migraine type.

Occasionally we allow a sleeping tablet or a tranquilizer, but patients should be told that while under treatment they need and may get less sleep. For instance, here in Italy where it is customary to sleep during the siesta which lasts from one to four in the afternoon most patients find that though they lie down they are unable to sleep.

"...severe sunburn always produces a temporary rise in weight, evidently due to water retention."

We encourage swimming and sun bathing during treatment, but it should be remembered that a severe sunburn always produces a temporary rise in weight, evidently due to water retention. The same may be seen when a patient gets a common cold during treatment. Finally, the weight can temporarily increase - paradoxical though this may sound - after an exceptional physical exertion of long duration leading to a feeling of exhaustion. A game of tennis, a vigorous swim, a run, a ride on horseback or a round of golf do not have this effect; but a long trek, a day of skiing, rowing or cycling or dancing into the small hours usually result in a gain of weight on the following day, unless the patient is in perfect training. In patients coming from abroad, where they always use their cars, we often see this effect after a strenuous day of shopping on foot, sightseeing and visits to galleries and museums. Though the extra muscular effort involved does consume some additional Calories, this appears to be offset by the retention of water which the tired circulation cannot at once eliminate.

"...this appears to be offset by the retention of water which the tired circulation cannot at once eliminate."

Appetite-reducing Drugs

We hardly ever use amphetamines, the appetite-reducing drugs such as Dexedrin, Dexamil, Preludin, etc., as there seems to be no need for them during the HCG treatment. The only time we find them useful is when a patient is, for impelling and unforeseen reasons, obliged to forego the injections for three to four days and yet wishes to continue the diet so that he need not interrupt the course.

Unforeseen Interruptions of Treatment

If an interruption of treatment lasting more than four days is necessary, the patient must increase his diet to at least 800 Calories by adding meat, eggs, cheese, and milk to his diet after the third day, as otherwise he will find himself so hungry and weak that he is unable to go about his usual occupation. If the interval lasts less than two weeks the patient can directly resume injections and the 500-Calorie diet, but if the interruption lasts longer he must again eat normally until he has had his third injection.

Section Five: **Dietary Errors & Other Factors**

When a patient knows beforehand that he will have to travel and be absent for more than four days, it is always better to stop injections three days before he is due to leave so that he can have the three days of strict dieting which are necessary after the last injection at home. This saves him from the almost impossible task of having to arrange the 500 Calorie diet while en route, and he can thus enjoy a much greater dietary freedom from the day of his departure. Interruptions occurring before 20 effective injections have been given are most undesirable, because with less than that number of injections some weight is liable to be regained. After the 20th injection an unavoidable interruption is merely a loss of time.

Muscular Fatigue

"...some patients complain that lifting a weight or climbing stairs requires a greater muscular effort than before."

Towards the end of a full course, when a good deal of fat has been rapidly lost, some patients complain that lifting a weight or climbing stairs requires a greater muscular effort than before. They feel neither breathlessness nor exhaustion but simply that their muscles have to work harder. This phenomenon, which disappears soon after the end of the treatment, is caused by the removal of abnormal fat deposited between, in, and around the muscles. The removal of this fat makes the muscles too long, and so in order to achieve a certain skeletal movement - say the bending of an arm - the muscles have to perform greater contraction than before. Within a short while the muscle adjusts itself perfectly to the new situation, but under HCG the loss of fat is so rapid that this adjustment cannot keep up with it. Patients often have to be reassured that this does not mean that they are "getting weak". This phenomenon does not occur in patients who regularly take vigorous exercise and continue to do so during treatment.

Massage Precautions

"...removal of this fat makes the muscles too long, and so in order to achieve a certain skeletal movement... the muscles have to perform greater contraction than before."

I never allow any kind of massage during treatment. It is entirely unnecessary and merely disturbs a very delicate process which is going on in the tissues. Few indeed are the masseurs and masseuses who can resist the temptation to knead and hammer abnormal fat deposits. In the course of rapid reduction it is sometimes possible to pick up a fold of skin which has not yet had time to adjust itself, as it always does under HCG, to the changed figure. This fold contains its normal subcutaneous fat and may be almost an inch thick. It is one of the main objects of the HCG treatment to keep that fat there. Patients and their masseurs do not always understand this and give this fat a working-over. I have seen such patients who were as black and blue as if they had received a sound thrashing.

In my opinion, massage, thumping, rolling, kneading, and shivering undertaken for the purpose of reducing abnormal fat can do nothing but harm. We once had the honor of treating the proprietress of a high class institution that specialized in such antics. She had the audacity to confess that she was taking our treatment to convince her clients of the efficacy of her methods, which she had found useless in her own case.

How anyone in his right mind is able to believe that fatty tissue can be shifted mechanically or be made to vanish by squeezing is beyond my comprehension. The only effect obtained is severe bruising. The torn tissue then forms scars, and these slowly contract making the fatty tissue even harder and more unyielding.

Section Five: Dietary Errors & Other Factors

"She had maintained both her weight and the improvement of her ankles."

A lady once consulted us for her most ungainly legs. Large masses of fat bulged over the ankles of her tiny feet, and there were about 40 lbs. too much on her hips and thighs. We assured her that this overweight could be lost and that her ankles would markedly improve in the process. Her treatment progressed most satisfactorily but to our surprise there was no improvement in her ankles. We then discovered that she had for years been taking every kind of mechanical, electric and heat treatment for her legs and that she had made up her mind to resort to plastic surgery if we failed.

Re-examining the fat above her ankles, we found that it was unusually hard. We attributed this to the countless minor injuries inflicted by kneading. These injuries had healed but had left a tough network of connective scar-tissue in which the fat was imprisoned. Ready to try anything, she was put to bed for the remaining three weeks of her first course with her lower legs tightly strapped in unyielding bandages. Every day the pressure was increased. The combination of HCG, diet and strapping brought about a marked improvement in the shape of her ankles. At the end of her first course she returned to her home abroad. Three months later she came back for her second course. She had maintained both her weight and the improvement of her ankles. The same procedure was repeated, and after five weeks she left the hospital with a normal weight and legs that, if not exactly shapely, were at least unobtrusive. Where no such injuries of the tissues have been inflicted by inappropriate methods of treatment, these drastic measures are never necessary.

Blood Sugar

"...it occasionally happens that the blood sugar drops below normal..."

Towards the end of a course or when a patient has nearly reached his normal weight it occasionally happens that the blood sugar drops below normal, and we have even seen this in patients who had an abnormally high blood sugar before treatment. Such an attack of hypoglycemia is almost identical with the one seen in diabetics who have taken too much insulin. The attack comes on suddenly; there is the same feeling of light-headedness, weakness in the knees, trembling, and unmotivated sweating; but under HCG, hypoglycemia does not produce any feeling of hunger. All these symptoms are almost instantly relieved by taking two heaped teaspoons of sugar.

"Some patients mistake the effects of emotional stress for hypoglycemia."

In the course of treatment the possibility of such an attack is explained to those patients who are in a phase in which a drop in blood sugar may occur. They are instructed to keep sugar or glucose sweets handy, particularly when driving a car. They are also told to watch the effect of taking sugar very carefully and report the following day. This is important, because anxious patients to whom such an attack has been explained are apt to take sugar unnecessarily, in which case it inevitably produces a gain in weight and does not dramatically relieve the symptoms for which it was taken, proving that these were not due to hypoglycemia. Some patients mistake the effects of emotional stress for hypoglycemia. When the symptoms are quickly relieved by sugar this is proof that they were indeed due to an abnormal lowering of the blood sugar, and in that case there is no increase in the weight on the following day. We always suggest that sugar be taken if the patient is in doubt.

Once such an attack has been relieved with sugar we have never seen it recur on the immediately subsequent days, and only very rarely does a patient have two such attacks separated by several days during a course of treatment. In patients who have not eaten sufficiently during the first two days of treatment we sometimes give sugar when the minor symptoms usually felt during the first three days of treatment continue beyond that time, and in some cases this has seemed to speed up the euphoria ordinarily associated with the HCG method.

Section Five: **Dietary Errors & Other Factors**

"At the beginning of treatment the change in measurements is somewhat greater..."

"Once HCG is in solution it is far less stable."

"...any brand made by a reliable pharmaceutical company is probably as good as any other."

The Ratio of Pounds to Inches

An interesting feature of the HCG method is that, regardless of how fat a patient is, the greatest circumference -- abdomen or hips as the case may be is reduced at a constant rate which is extraordinarily close to 1 cm. per kilogram of weight lost. At the beginning of treatment the change in measurements is somewhat greater than this, but at the end of a course it is almost invariably found that the girth is as many centimeters less as the number of kilograms by which the weight has been reduced. I have never seen this clear cut relationship in patients that try to reduce by dieting only.

Preparing the Solution

Human chorionic gonadotrophin comes on the market as a highly soluble powder which is the pure substance extracted from the urine of pregnant women. Such preparations are carefully standardized, and any brand made by a reliable pharmaceutical company is probably as good as any other. The substance should be extracted from the urine and not from the placenta, and it must of course be of human and not of animal origin. The powder is sealed in ampoules or in rubber-capped bottles in varying amounts which are stated in International Units. In this form HCG is stable; however, only such preparations should be used that have the date of manufacture and the date of expiry clearly stated on the label or package. A suitable solvent is always supplied in a separate ampoule in the same package.

Once HCG is in solution it is far less stable. It may be kept at room-temperature for two to three days, but if the solution must be kept longer it should always be refrigerated. When treating only one or two cases simultaneously, vials containing a small number of units say 1000 I.U. should be used. The 10 cc. of solvent which is supplied by the manufacturer is injected into the rubber- capped bottle containing the HCG, and the powder must dissolve instantly. Of this solution 1.25 cc. are withdrawn for each injection. One such bottle of 1000 I.U. therefore furnishes 8 injections. When more than one patient is being treated, they should not each have their own bottle but rather all be injected from the same vial and a fresh solution made when this is empty.

As we are usually treating a fair number of patients at the same time, we prefer to use vials containing 5000 units. With these the manufactures also supply 10 cc. of solvent. Of such a solution 0.25 cc. contain the 125 I.U., which is the standard dose for all cases and which should never be exceeded. This small amount is awkward to handle accurately (it requires an insulin syringe) and is wasteful, because there is a loss of solution in the nozzle of the syringe and in the needle. We therefore prefer a higher dilution, which we prepare in the following way: The solvent supplied is injected into the rubbercapped bottle containing the 5000 I.U . As these bottles are too small to hold more solvent, we withdraw 5 cc., inject it into an empty rubber-capped bottle and add 5 cc. of normal saline to each bottle. This gives us 10 cc. of solution in each bottle, and of this solution 0.5 cc. contains 125 I.U. This amount is convenient to inject with an ordinary syringe.

Injecting HCG & Tissue Reaction

HCG produces little or no tissue-reaction, it is completely painless and in the many thousands of injections we have given we have never seen an inflammatory or suppurative reaction at the site of the injection.

Section Five: **Dietary Errors & Other Factors**

One should avoid leaving a vacuum in the bottle after preparing the solution or after withdrawal of the amount required for the injections as otherwise alcohol used for sterilizing a frequently perforated rubber cap might be drawn into the solution. When sharp needles are used, it sometimes happens that a little bit of rubber is punched out of the rubber cap and can be seen as a small black speck floating in the solution. As these bits of rubber are heavier than the solution they rapidly settle out, and it is thus easy to avoid drawing them into the syringe.

"There are hardly any contraindications to the HCG method."

We use very fine needles that are two inches long and inject deep intragluteally in the outer upper quadrant of the buttocks. The injection should if possible not be given into the superficial fat layers, which in very obese patients must be compressed so as to enable the needle to reach the muscle. Obviously needles and syringes must be carefully washed, sterilized and handled aseptically.[8] It is also important that the daily injection should be given at intervals as close to 24 hours as possible. Any attempt to economize in time by giving larger doses at longer intervals is doomed to produce less satisfactory results.

There are hardly any contraindications to the HCG method. Treatment can be continued in the presence of abscesses, suppuration, large infected wounds and major fractures. Surgery and general anesthesia are no reason to stop and we have given treatment during a severe attack of malaria. Acne or boils are no contraindication; the former usually clears up, and furunculosis comes to an end. Thrombophlebitis is no contraindication, and we have treated several obese patients with HCG and the 500-Calorie diet while suffering from this condition. Our impression has been that in obese patients the phlebitis does rather better and certainly no worse than under the usual treatment alone. This also applies to patients suffering from varicose ulcers which tend to heal rapidly.

"...uterine fibroids seem to be in no way affected by HCG in the doses we use..."

Fibroids & HCG

While uterine fibroids seem to be in no way affected by HCG in the doses we use, we have found that very large, externally palpable uterine myomas are apt to give trouble. We are convinced that this is entirely due to the rather sudden disappearance of fat from the pelvic bed upon which they rest and that it is the weight of the tumor pressing on the underlying tissues which accounts for the discomfort or pain which may arise during treatment. While we disregard even fair-sized or multiple myomas, we insist that very large ones be operated before treatment. We have had patients present themselves for reducing fat from their abdomen who showed no signs of obesity, but had a large abdominal tumor.

Gallstones

"This may be due to the almost complete absence of fat from the diet..."

Small stones in the gall bladder may in patients who have recently had typical colics cause more frequent colics under treatment with HCG. This may be due to the almost complete absence of fat from the diet, which prevents the normal emptying of the gall bladder. Before undertaking treatment we explain to such patients that there is a risk of more frequent and possibly severe symptoms and that it may become necessary to operate. If they are prepared to take this risk and provided they agree to undergo an operation if we consider this imperative, we proceed with treatment, as after weight reduction with HCG the operative risk is considerably reduced in an obese patient. In such cases we always give a drug which stimulates the flow of bile, and in the majority of cases nothing untoward happens. On the other hand, we have looked for and not found any evidence to suggest that the HCG treatment leads to the formation of gallstones as pregnancy sometimes does.

The Heart

"...many such patients are referred to us by cardiologists."

Disorders of the heart are not as a rule contraindications. In fact, the removal of abnormal fat - particularly from the heart-muscle and from the surrounding of the coronary arteries - can only be beneficial in cases of myocardial weakness, and many such patients are referred to us by cardiologists. Within the first week of treatment all patients - not only heart cases - remark that they have lost much of their breathlessness.

Coronary Occlusion

"...treatment is then started under careful control and it is usual to find a further electrocardiographic improvement..."

In obese patients who have recently survived a coronary occlusion, we adopt the following procedure in collaboration with the cardiologist. We wait until no further electrocardiographic changes have occurred for a period of three months. Routine treatment is then started under careful control and it is usual to find a further electrocardiographic improvement of a condition which was previously stationary.

In the thousands of cases we have treated we have not once seen any sort of coronary incident occur during or shortly after treatment. The same applies to cerebral vascular accidents. Nor have we ever seen a case of thrombosis of any sort develop during treatment, even though a high blood pressure is rapidly lowered. In this respect, too, the HCG treatment resembles pregnancy.

Teeth and Vitamins

"...sometimes get more trouble under prolonged treatment..."

Patients whose teeth are in poor repair sometimes get more trouble under prolonged treatment, just as may occur in pregnancy. In such cases we do allow calcium and vitamin D, though not in an oily solution. The only other vitamin we permit is vitamin C, which we use in large doses combined with an antihistamine at the onset of a common cold. There is no objection to the use of an antibiotic if this is required, for instance by the dentist. In cases of bronchial asthma and hay fever we have occasionally resorted to cortisone during treatment and find that triamcinolone is the least likely to interfere with the loss of weight, but many asthmatics improve with HCG alone.

Alcohol & Alcoholism

"Obese heavy drinkers, even those bordering on alcoholism, often do surprisingly well under HCG."

Obese heavy drinkers, even those bordering on alcoholism, often do surprisingly well under HCG and it is exceptional for them to take a drink while under treatment. When they do, they find that a relatively small quantity of alcohol produces intoxication. Such patients say that they do not feel the need to drink. This may in part be due to the euphoria which the treatment produces and in part to the complete absence of the need for quick sustenance from which most obese patients suffer.

Though we have had a few cases that have continued abstinence long after treatment, others relapse as soon as they are back on a normal diet. We have a few "regular customers" who, having once been reduced to their normal weight, start to drink again though watching their weight. Then after some months they purposely overeat in order

Section Five: **Dietary Errors & Other Factors**

to gain sufficient weight for another course of HCG which temporarily gets them out of their drinking routine. We do not particularly welcome such cases, but we see no reason for refusing their request.

Tuberculosis

"...obese patients suffering from inactive pulmonary tuberculosis can be safely treated."

It is interesting that obese patients suffering from inactive pulmonary tuberculosis can be safely treated. We have under very careful control treated patients as early as three months after they were pronounced inactive and have never seen a relapse occur during or shortly after treatment. In fact, we only have one case on our records in which active tuberculosis developed in a young man about one year after a treatment which had lasted three weeks. Earlier X-rays showed a calcified spot from a childhood infection which had not produced clinical symptoms. There was a family history of tuberculosis, and his illness started under adverse conditions which certainly had nothing to do with the treatment. Residual calcifications from an early infection are exceedingly common, and we never consider them a contraindication to treatment.

The Painful Heel

In obese patients who have been trying desperately to keep their weight down by severe dieting, a curious symptom sometimes occurs. They complain of an unbearable pain in their heels which they feel only while standing or walking. As soon as they take the weight off their heels the pain ceases. These cases are the bane of the rheumatologists and orthopedic surgeons who have treated them before they come to us. All the usual investigations are entirely negative, and there is not the slightest response to anti- rheumatic medication or physiotherapy. The pain may be so severe that the patients are obliged to give up their occupation, and they are not infrequently labeled as a case of hysteria. When their heels are carefully examined one finds that the sole is softer than normal and that the heel bone - the calcaneus - can be distinctly felt, which is not the case in a normal foot.

"In both cases the pain completely disappears in 10-20 days of dieting..."

We interpret the condition as a lack of the hard fatty pad on which the calcaneus rests and which protects both the bone and the skin of the sole from pressure. This fat is like a springy cushion which carries the weight of the body. Standing on a heel in which this fat is missing or reduced must obviously be very painful. In their efforts to keep their weight down these patients have consumed this normal structural fat.

Those patients who have a normal or subnormal weight while showing the typically obese fat deposits are made to eat to capacity, often much against their will, for one week. They gain weight rapidly but there is no improvement in the painful heels. They are then started on the routine HCG treatment. Overweight patients are treated immediately. In both cases the pain completely disappears in 10-20 days of dieting, usually around the 15th day of treatment, and so far no case has had a relapse though we have been able to follow up such patients for years.

We are particularly interested in these cases, as they furnish further proof of the contention that HCG + 500 Calories not only removes abnormal fat but actually permits normal fat to be replaced, in spite of the deficient food intake. It is certainly not so that the mere loss of weight reduces the pain, because it frequently disappears before the weight the patient had prior to the period of forced feeding is reached.

Section Five: **Concluding HCG & Course Corrections**

The Skeptical Patient

Any doctor who starts using the HCG method for the first time will have considerable difficulty, particularly if he himself is not fully convinced, in making patients believe that they will not feel hungry on 500 Calories and that their face will not collapse. New patients always anticipate the phenomena they know so well from previous treatments and diets and are incredulous when told that these will not occur. We overcome all this by letting new patients spend a little time in the waiting room with older hands, who can always be relied upon to allay these fears with evangelistic zeal, often demonstrating the finer points on their own body.

A waiting-room filled with obese patients who congregate daily is a sort of group therapy. They compare notes and pop back into the waiting room after the consultation to announce the score of the last 24 hours to an enthralled audience. They cross-check on their diets and sometimes confess sins which they try to hide from us, usually with the result that the patient in whom they have confided palpitatingly tattles the whole disgraceful story to us with a "But don't let her know I told you."

Concluding an HCG Course

When the three days of dieting after the last injection are over, the patients are told that they may now eat anything they please, except sugar and starch provided they faithfully observe one simple rule. This rule is that they must have their own portable bathroom-scale always at hand, particularly while traveling. They must without fail weigh themselves every morning as they get out of bed, having first emptied their bladder. If they are in the habit of having breakfast in bed, they must weigh before breakfast. It takes about 3 weeks before the weight reached at the end of the treatment becomes stable, i.e. does not show violent fluctuations after an occasional excess. During this period patients must realize that the so-called carbohydrates, that is sugar, rice, bread, potatoes, pastries, etc, are by far the most dangerous. If no carbohydrates whatsoever are eaten, fats can be indulged in somewhat more liberally and even small quantities of alcohol, such as a glass of wine with meals, does no harm, but as soon as fats and starch are combined things are very liable to get out of hand. This has to be observed very carefully during the first 3 weeks after the treatment is ended otherwise disappointments are almost sure to occur.

Skipping a Meal: A 'Steak Day.'

As long as their weight stays within two pounds of the weight reached on the day of the last injection, patients should take no notice of any increase but the moment the scale goes beyond two pounds, even if this is only a few ounces, they must on that same day entirely skip breakfast and lunch but take plenty to drink. In the evening they must eat a huge steak with only an apple or a raw tomato. Of course this rule applies only to the morning weight. Ex-obese patients should never check their weight during the day, as there may be wide fluctuations and these are merely alarming and confusing.

It is of utmost importance that the meal is skipped on the same day as the scale registers an increase of more than two pounds and that missing the meals is not postponed until the following day. If a meal is skipped on the day in which a gain is registered in the morning this brings about an immediate drop of often over a pound.

"...making patients believe that they will not feel hungry on 500 Calories and that their face will not collapse."

"...patients are told that they may now eat anything they please, except sugar and starch..."

"This has to be observed very carefully during the first 3 weeks..."

Section Five: **Concluding HCG & Course Corrections**

But if the skipping of the meal - and skipping means literally skipping, not just having a light meal - is postponed the phenomenon does not occur and several days of strict dieting may be necessary to correct the situation.

Most patients hardly ever need to skip a meal. If they have eaten a heavy lunch they feel no desire to eat their dinner, and in this case no increase takes place. If they keep their weight at the point reached at the end of the treatment, even a heavy dinner does not bring about an increase of two pounds on the next morning and does not therefore call for any special measures. Most patients are surprised how small their appetite has become and yet how much they can eat without gaining weight. They no longer suffer from an abnormal appetite and feel satisfied with much less food than before. In fact, they are usually disappointed that they cannot manage their first normal meal, which they have been planning for weeks.

"Most patients are surprised how small their appetite has become and yet how much they can eat..."

Losing more Weight

An ex-patient should never gain more than two pounds without immediately correcting this, but it is equally undesirable that more than two lbs. be lost after treatment, because a greater loss is always achieved at the expense of normal fat. Any normal fat that is lost is invariably regained as soon as more food is taken, and it often happens that this rebound overshoots the upper two pound limit.

"...it is equally undesirable that more than two lbs. be lost after treatment..."

Trouble After Treatment: Two Areas of Difficulty

Two difficulties may be encountered in the immediate post-treatment period. When a patient has consumed all his abnormal fat or, when after a full course, the injection has temporarily lost its efficacy owing to the body having gradually evolved a counter regulation, the patient at once begins to feel much more hungry and even weak. In spite of repeated warnings, some over-enthusiastic patients do not report this. However, in about two days the fact that they are being undernourished becomes visible in their faces, and treatment is then stopped at once. In such cases - and only in such cases - we allow a very slight increase in the diet, such as an extra apple, 150 grams of meat or two or three extra breadsticks during the three days of dieting after the last injection.

"...it is impossible to reduce a patient, however enthusiastic, beyond his normal weight."

When abnormal fat is no longer being put into circulation either because it has been consumed or because immunity has set in, this is always felt by the patient as sudden, intolerable and constant hunger. In this sense, the HCG method is completely self-limiting. With HCG it is impossible to reduce a patient, however enthusiastic, beyond his normal weight. As soon as no more abnormal fat is being issued, the body starts consuming normal fat, and this is always regained as soon as ordinary feeding is resumed. The patient then finds that the 2-3 lbs. he has lost during the last days of treatment are immediately regained. A meal is skipped and maybe a pound is lost. The next day this pound is regained, in spite of a careful watch over the food intake. In a few days a tearful patient is back in the consulting room, convinced that her case is a failure.

All that is happening is that the essential fat lost at the end of the treatment, owing to the patient's reluctance to report a much greater hunger, is being replaced. The weight at which such a patient must stabilize thus lies 2-3 lbs. higher than the weight reached at the end of the treatment. Once this higher basic level is established, further difficulties in controlling the weight at the new point of stabilization hardly arise.

Section Five: **Concluding HCG & Course Corrections**

Beware of Over-enthusiasm

"They disregard the advice to eat anything they please except sugar and starch and want to play safe."

The other trouble which is frequently encountered immediately after treatment is again due to over-enthusiasm. Some patients cannot believe that they can eat fairly normally without regaining weight. They disregard the advice to eat anything they please except sugar and starch and want to play safe. They try more or less to continue the 500-Calorie diet on which they felt so well during treatment and make only minor variations, such as replacing the meat with an egg, cheese, or a glass of milk. To their horror they find that in spite of this bravura, their weight goes up. So, following instructions, they skip one meager lunch and at night eat only a little salad and drink a pot of unsweetened tea, becoming increasingly hungry and weak. The next morning they find that they have increased yet another pound. They feel terrible, and even the dreaded swelling of their ankles is back. Normally we check our patients one week after they have been eating freely, but these cases return in a few days. Either their eyes are filled with tears or they angrily imply that when we told them to eat normally we were just fooling them.

Protein Deficiency Weight Gain

"Unless an adequate amount of protein is eaten as soon as the treatment is over, protein deficiency is bound to develop..."

Here too, the explanation is quite simple. During treatment the patient has been only just above the verge of protein deficiency and has had the advantage of protein being fed back into his system from the breakdown of fatty tissue. Once the treatment is over there is no more HCG in the body and this process no longer takes place. Unless an adequate amount of protein is eaten as soon as the treatment is over, protein deficiency is bound to develop, and this inevitably causes the marked retention of water known as hunger-edema.

The treatment is very simple. The patient is told to eat two eggs for breakfast and a huge steak for lunch and dinner followed by a large helping of cheese and to phone through the weight the next morning. When these instructions are followed a stunned voice is heard to report that two lbs. have vanished overnight, that the ankles are normal but that sleep was disturbed, owing to an extraordinary need to pass large quantities of water. The patient having learned this lesson usually has no further trouble.

Relapses & Permanent Weight Loss

"...one can say that 60%-70% of our cases experience little or no difficulty in holding their weight permanently."

As a general rule one can say that 60%-70% of our cases experience little or no difficulty in holding their weight permanently. Relapses may be due to negligence in the basic rule of daily weighing. Many patients think that this is unnecessary and that they can judge any increase from the fit of their clothes. Some do not carry their scale with them on a journey as it is cumbersome and takes a big bite out of their luggage-allowance when flying. This is a disastrous mistake, because after a course of HCG as much as 10 lbs. can be regained without any noticeable change in the fit of the clothes. The reason for this is that after treatment newly acquired fat is at first evenly distributed and does not show the former preference for certain parts of the body.

Pregnancy or the menopause may annul the effect of a previous treatment. Women who take treatment during the one year after the last menstruation - that is at the onset of the menopause - do just as well as others, but among them the relapse rate is higher until the menopause is fully established. The period of one year after the last menstruation applies only to women who are not being treated with ovarian hormones.

If these are taken, the premenopausal period may be indefinitely prolonged. Late teenage girls who suffer from attacks of compulsive eating have by far the worst record of all as far as relapses are concerned.

Patients who have once taken the treatment never seem to hesitate to come back for another short course as soon as they notice that their weight is once again getting out of hand. They come quite cheerfully and hopefully, assured that they can be helped again. Repeat courses are often even more satisfactory than the first treatment and have the advantage, as do second courses, that the patient already, knows that he will feel comfortable throughout.

Plan of a Normal Course (Utilizing Injections)

125 I.U. of HCG daily (except during menstruation) until 40 injections have been given.

Until 3rd injection forced feeding.

After 3rd injection, 500 Calorie diet to be continued until 72 hours after the last injection.

For the following 3 weeks, all foods allowed except starch and sugar in any form (careful with very sweet fruit).

After 3 weeks, very gradually add starch in small quantities, always controlled by morning weighing.

"Repeat courses are often even more satisfactory than the first treatment and have the advantage, as do second courses, that the patient already, knows that he will feel comfortable throughout."

CONCLUSIONS: The HCG + 500 Calorie Diet Method

"The HCG + diet method can bring relief to every case of obesity, but the method is not simple."

The HCG + diet method can bring relief to **every** case of obesity, but the method is **not simple**. It is very time consuming and requires perfect **cooperation** between physician and patient. Each case must be handled individually, and **the physician** must have time to answer questions, allay fears and remove misunderstandings. He must also check the patient daily. When something goes wrong he must at once investigate until he finds the reason for any gain that may have occurred. **In most cases it is useless to hand the patient a diet-sheet and let the nurse give him a "shot."**

The method involves a **highly complex bodily mechanism**, and even though our theory may be wrong the physician must make himself some sort of picture of what is actually happening; otherwise he will **not** be able to deal with such difficulties as may arise during treatment.

"...adhere very strictly to the technique and the interpretations here outlined..."

I must beg those trying the method for the first time to **adhere very strictly** to the **technique** and the **interpretations** here outlined and thus treat a few hundred cases before embarking on experiments of their own, and until then **refrain** from introducing innovations, however thrilling they may seem. In a new method, innovations or departures from the original technique can only be usefully evaluated against a substantial background of experience with what is at the moment the orthodox procedure.

I have tried to cover all the problems that come to my mind. Yet a bewildering array of new questions keep arising, and my interpretations are still fluid. In particular, I have never had an opportunity of conducting the laboratory investigations which are so necessary for a theoretical understanding of clinical observations, and I can only hope that those more fortunately placed will in time be able to fill this gap.

"...our world will be a happier place for countless fellow men and women."

The **problems of obesity** are perhaps not so dramatic as the problems of cancer, or polio, but they often cause life long suffering. How many promising careers have been ruined by excessive fat; how many lives have been shortened. If some way -however cumbersome - can be found to cope effectively with this universal problem of modern civilized man, our world will be a happier place for countless fellow men and women.

GLOSSARY & ADDENDUM

GLOSSRY & ADDENDUM

Section Five: Dr. Simeons Glossary of Terms:

Acne
Common skin disease in which pimples, often containing pus, appear on face, neck and shoulders.

ACTH
Abbreviation for adrenocorticotrophic hormone. One of the many hormones produced by the anterior lobe of the pituitary gland. ACTH controls the outer part, rind or cortex of the adrenal glands. When ACTH is injected it dramatically relieves arthritic pain, but it has many undesirable side effects, among which is a condition similar to severe obesity. ACTH is now usually replaced by cortisone.

Adrenalin
Hormone produced by the inner part of the Adrenals. Among many other functions, adrenalin is concerned with blood pressure, emotional stress, fear and cold.

Adrenals
Endocrine glands. Small bodies situated atop the kidneys and hence also known as suprarenal glands. The adrenals have an outer rind or cortex which produces vitally important hormones, among which are Cortisone similar substances. The adrenal cortex is controlled by ACTH. The inner part of the adrenals, the medulla, secretes adrenalin and is chiefly controlled by the autonomous nervous system.

Adrenocortex
See adrenals.

Amphetamines
Synthetic drugs which reduce the awareness of hunger and stimulate mental activity, rendering sleep impossible. When used for the latter two purposes they are dangerously habit-forming. They do not diminish the body's need for food, but merely suppress the perception of that need. The original drug was known as Benzedrine, from which modern variants such as Dexedrine, Dexamil, and Preludin, etc., have been derived. Amphetamines may help an obese patient to prevent a further increase in weight but are unsatisfactory for reducing, as they do not cure the underlying disorder and as their prolonged use may lead to malnutrition and addiction.

Arteriosclerosis
Hardening of the arterial wall through the calcification of abnormal deposits of a fatlike substance known as cholesterol.

Aschhieim-Zondek
Authors of a test by which early pregnancy can be diagnosed by injecting a woman's urine into female mice. The HCG present in pregnancy urine produces certain changes in the vagina of these animals. Many similar tests, using other animals such as rabbits, frogs, etc. have been devised.

Assimilate
Absorb digested food from the intestines.

Autonomous
Here used to describe the independent or vegetative nervous system which manages the automatic regulations of the body.

Basal Metabolism
The body's chemical turnover at complete rest and when fasting. The basal metabolic rate is expressed as the amount of oxygen used up in a given time. The basal metabolic rate (BMR) is controlled by the thyroid gland.

Calorie
The physicist's calorie is the amount of heat required to raise the temperature of 1 cc. of water by 1 degree Centigrade. The dieticiari's Calorie (always written with a capital C) is 1000 times greater. Thus when we speak of a 500 Calorie diet this means that the body is being supplied with as much fuel as would be required to raise the temperature of 500 liters of water by 1 degree Centigrade or 50 liters by 10 degrees. This

Section Five: Dr. Simeons Glossary of Terms:

is quite insufficient to cover the heat and energy requirements of an adult body. In the HCG method the deficit is made up from the abnormal fat-deposits, of which 1 lb. furnishes the body with more than 2000 Calories. As this is roughly the amount lost every day, a patient under HCG is never short of fuel.

Cerebral

Of the brain. Cerebral vascular disease is a disorder concerning the blood vessels of the brain, such as cerebral thrombosis or hemorrhage, known as apoplexy or stroke.

Cholesterol

A fatlike substance contained in almost every cell of the body. In the blood it exists in two forms, known as free and esterified. The latter form is under certain conditions deposited in the inner lining of the arteries (see arteriosclerosis). No clear and definite relationship between fat intake and cholesterol-level in the blood has yet been established.

Chorionic

Of the chorion, which is part of the placenta or after-birth. The term chorionic is justly applied to HCG, as this hormone is exclusively produced in the placenta, from where it enters the human mother's blood and is later excreted in her urine.

Compulsive Eating

A form of oral gratification with which a repressed sex-instinct is sometimes vicariously relieved. Compulsive eating must not be confused with the real hunger from which most obese patients suffer.

Congenital

Any condition which exists at or before birth.

Coronary Arteries

Two blood vessels which encircle the heart and supply all the blood required by the heart-muscle.

Corpus Luteum

A yellow body which forms in the ovary at the follicle from which an egg has been detached. This body acts as an endocrine gland and plays an important role in menstruation and pregnancy. Its secretion is one of the sex hormones, and it is stimulated by another hormone known as LSH, which stands for luteum stimulating hormones. LSH is produced in the anterior lobe of the pituitary gland. LSH is truly gonadotrophic and must never be confused with HCG, which is a totally different substance, having no direct action on the corpus luteum.

Cortex

Outer covering or rind. The term is applied to the outer part of the adrenals but is also used to describe the gray matter which covers the white matter of the brain.

Cortisone

A synthetic substance which acts like an adrenal hormone. It is today used in the treatment of a large number of illnesses, and several chemical variants have been produced, among which are prednisone and triamcinolone.

Cushing

A great American brain surgeon who described a condition of extreme obesity associated with symptoms of adrenal disorder. Cushing's Syndrome may be caused by organic disease of the pituitary or the adrenal glands but, as was later discovered, it also occurs as a result of excessive ACTH medication.

Diencephalon

A primitive and hence very old part of the brain which lies between and under the two large hemispheres. In man the diencephalon (or hypothalamus) is subordinate to the higher brain or cortex, and yet it ultimately controls all that happens inside the body. It regulates all the endocrine glands, the autonomous nervous system, the turnover

Section Five: Dr. Simeons Glossary of Terms:

of fat and sugar. It seems also to be the seat of the primitive animal instincts and is the relay station at which emotions are translated into bodily reactions.

Diuretic — Any substance that increases the flow of urine.

Dysfunction — Abnormal functioning of any organ, be this excessive, deficient or in any way altered.

Edema — An abnormal accumulation of water in the tissues.

Electrocardiogram — Tracing of electric phenomena taking place in the heart during each beat. The tracing provides information about the condition and working of the heart which is not otherwise obtainable.

Endocrine — We distinguish endocrine and exocrine glands. The former produce hormones, chemical regulators, which they secrete directly into the blood circulation in the gland and from where they are carried all over the body. Examples of endocrine glands are the pituitary, the thyroid and the adrenals. Exocrine glands produce a visible secretion such as saliva, sweat, urine. There are also glands which are endocrine and exocrine. Examples are the testicles, the prostate and the pancreas, which produces the hormone insulin and digestive ferments which flow from the gland into the intestinal tract. Endocrine glands are closely inter dependent of each other, they are linked to the autonomous nervous system and the diencephalon presides over this whole incredibly complex regulatory system.

Emaciated — Grossly undernourished.

Euphoria — A feeling of particular physical and mental well being.

Feral — Wild, unrestrained.

Fibroid — Any benign new growth of connective tissue. When such a tumor originates from a muscle, it is known as a myoma. The most common seat of myomas is the uterus.

Follicle — Any small bodily cyst or sac containing a liquid. Here the term applies to the ovarian cyst in which the egg is formed. The egg is expelled when a ripe follicle bursts and this is known as ovulation (see corpus luteurn).

FSH — Abbreviation for follicle-stimulating hormone. FSH is another (see corpus luteum) anterior pituitary hormone which acts directly on the ovarian follicle and is therefore correctly called a gonadotrophin.

Glands — See endocrine.

Gonadotrophin — See corpus luteum, follicle and FSH. Gonadotrophic literally means sex gland-directed. FSH, LSH and the equivalent hormones in the male, all produced in the anterior lobe of the pituitary gland, are true gonadotrophins. Unfortunately and confusingly, the term gonadotrophin has also been applied to the placental hormone of pregnancy known as human chorionic gonadotrophin (HCG). This hormone acts on the diencephalon and can only indirectly influence the sex-glands via the anterior lobe of the pituitary.

Section Five: Dr. Simeons Glossary of Terms:

HCG Abbreviation for human chorionic gonadotrophin

Hormones See endocrine.

Hypertension High blood pressure.

Hypoglycemia A condition in which the blood sugar is below normal. It can be relieved by eating sugar.

Hypophysis Another name for the pituitary gland.

Hypothesis A tentative explanation or speculation on how observed facts and isolated scientific data can be brought into an intellectually satisfying relationship of cause and effect. Useful for directing further research, but not necessarily an exposition of what is believed to be the truth. Before a hypothesis can advance to the dignity of a theory or a law, it must be confirmed by all future research. As soon as research turns up data which no longer fit the hypothesis, it is immediately abandoned for a better one.

LSH See corpus luteum.

Metabolism See basal metabolism.

Migraine Severe half-sided headache often associated with vomiting.

Mucoid Slime-like.

Myocardium The heart-muscle.

Myoma See fibroid.

Myxedema Accumulation of a mucoid substance in the tissues which occurs in cases of severe primary thyroid deficiency.

Neolithic In the history of human culture we distinguish the Early Stone Age or Paleolithic, the Middle Stone Age or Mesolithic and the New Stone Age or Neolithic period. The Neolithic period started about 8000 years ago when the first attempts at agriculture, pottery and animal domestication made at the end of the Mesolithic period suddenly began to develop rapidly along the road that led to modern civilization.

Normal Saline A low concentration of salt in water equal to the salinity of body fluids.

Phlebitis An inflammation of the veins. When a blood-clot forms at the site of the inflammation, we speak of thrombophlebitis.

Pituitary A very complex endocrine gland which lies at the base of the skull, consisting chiefly of an anterior and a posterior lobe. The pituitary is controlled by the diencephalon, which regulates the anterior lobe by means of hormones which reach it through small blood vessels. The posterior lobe is controlled by nerves which run from the diencephalon into this part of the gland. The anterior lobe secretes many hormones, among which are those that regulate other glands such as the thyroid, the adrenals and the sex glands.

Section Five: Dr. Simeons Glossary of Terms:

Placenta
The after-birth. In women, a large and highly complex organ through which the child in the womb receives its nourishment from the mother's body. It is the organ in which HCG is manufactured and then given off into the mother's blood.

Protein
The living substance in plant and animal cells. Herbivorous animals can thrive on plant protein alone, but man must have some protein of animal origin (milk, eggs or flesh) to live healthily. When insufficient protein is eaten, the body retains water.

Psoriasis
A skin disease which produces scaly patches. These tend to disappear during pregnancy and during the treatment of obesity by the HCG method.

Renal
Of the kidney.

Reserpine
An Indian drug extensively used in the treatment of high blood pressure and some forms of mental disorder.

Retention Enema
The slow infusion of a liquid into the rectum, from where it is absorbed and not evacuated.

Sacrum
A fusion of the lower vertebrate into the large bony mass to which the pelvis is attached.

Sedimentation Rate
The speed at which a suspension of red blood cells settles out. A rapid settling out is called a high sedimentation rate and may be indicative of a large number of bodily disorders of pregnancy.

Sexual Selection
A sexual preference for individuals which show certain traits. If this preference or selection goes on generation after generation, more and more individuals showing the trait will appear among the general population. The natural environment has little or nothing to do with this process. Sexual selection therefore differs from natural selection, to which modern man is no longer subject because he changes his environment rather than let the environment change him.

Striation
Tearing of the lower layers of the skin owing to rapid stretching in obesity or during pregnancy. When first formed striae are dark reddish lines which later change into white scars.

Suprarenal Glands
See adrenals.

Syndrome
A group of symptoms which in their association are characteristic of a particular disorder.

Thrombophlebitis
See phlebitis.

Thrombus
A blood-clot in a blood-vessel.

Triamcinolone
A modern derivative of cortisone.

Uric Acid
A product of incomplete protein-breakdown or utilization in the body. When uric acid becomes deposited in the gristle of the joints we speak of gout.

Section Five: Dr. Simeons Glossary of Terms:

Varicose Ulcers   Chronic ulceration above the ankles due to varicose veins which interfere with the normal blood circulation in the affected areas.

Vegetative   See autonomous.

Vertebrate   Any animal that has a back-bone.

Section Five: Addendum & Footnotes

ADDENDUM: Literary References to the Use of Chorionic Gonadotrophin In Obesity

THE LANCET

Nov. 6, 1954	Article	Simeons
Nov. 15, 1958	Letter to Editor	Simeons
July 29, 1961	Letter to Editor	Lebon
Dec. 9, 1961	Article	Carne
Dec. 9, 1961	Letter to Editor	Kalina
Jan. 6, 1962	Letter to Editor	Simeons
Nov. 26, 1966	Letter to Editor	Lebon

THE JOURNAL OF THE AMERICAN GERIATRIC SOCIETY

Jan. 1956	Article	Simeons
Oct. 1964	Article	Harris& Warsaw
Feb. 1966	Article	Lebon

THE AMERICAN JOURNAL OF CLINICAL NUTRITION

Sept.-Oct. 1959	Article	Sohar
March 1963	Article	Craig et al.
Sept. 1963	Letter to Editor	Simeons
March 1964	Article	Frank
Sept. 1964	Letter to Editor	Simeons
Feb. 1965	Letter to Editor	Hutton
June 1969	Editorial	Albrink
June 1969	Special Article	Gusman

THE JOURNAL OF PLASTIC SURGERY (British)

| April 1962 | Article | Lebon |

THE SOUTH AFRICAN MEDICAL JOURNAL

| Feb 1963 | Article | Politzer,Berson & Flaks |

A.T.W. SIMEONS POUNDS AND INCHES
Salvator Mundi International Hospital, Rome, Italy

VETSUCHT (Netherlands Edition) Wetenschappelijke Uitgeverij, N.V. Amsterdam

MAN'S PRESUMPTUOUS BRAIN Longman's, Green, London
E.P. Dutton, New York (hardback) Dutton Paperbacks, New York

Section Five: Addendum & Footnotes

**FOOTNOTES
&
REFERENCES**

[1]   A list of references to the more important articles is given at the end of this booklet.

[2]   "Current account" is the British name for what Americans call a checking account.

[3]   There is some clinical evidence to suggest that those symptoms of Cushing's Syndrome which resemble true obesity are caused by the same mechanism which causes common obesity, while the other symptoms of the syndrome are directly due to adrenocortical dysfunction.

[4]   World War II.

[5]   Confinement = the concluding state of pregnancy

[6]   As we are speaking of purely regulatory disorders, we obviously exclude all such cases in which there are gross organic lesions of the pituitary or of the sex-glands themselves.

[7]   We use 1 tablet of hygroton.

[8]   This practice is obsolete. Modern sanitary methods dictate throwing away used needles and syringes and using new ones for each injection.

[9]   Wherever unfamiliar terms are used, they will be found in their respective alphabetical place in the 'Glossary of Terms.'

**SUMMARY OF
GRAPHIC
& LAYOUT
ADDITIONS**

We have respectfully added the following copyrighted design and layout features:

Table of Contents.
Bold emphasis for illumination, emphasis and clarification.
Side bar 'highlighted quotes' of important comments.
Reverse bold headlines for easier navigation.
Addition of several Tables and Graphics for clarification of concepts.

Section Six:

'A Tangled WEB... Untangled.'

> *"No end of injustice is done to obese patients by accusing them of compulsive eating..."*
>
> *Dr. A.T.W. Simeons*

Defeat OBESITY...Forever!

The HCG Assisted 500 Calorie Weight Loss Cure

Section Six: **A Tangled Web**

"In my opinion the HCG diet protocol is not a do-it-yourself kit."

"They are more interested in treating the symptoms and selling supplements and multiple medications to the chronically obese... than curing them forever."

Said the Spider to the Fly...

Here's **something that concerns me**. It is a **justified** and **ethical** concern.

On the **web** you will find **all kinds** of HCG offers. Some of them offering to sell you 'direct without a prescription' HCG and a variety of other products. In my opinion the HCG diet protocol is **not a do-it-yourself** kit. It is meant to be **physician** directed.

I don't know who these people are. Some of them are probably sincere and have the best of intentions for you. To others you are just **their prey**. Don't be.

The **HCG + 500C** plan is a legitimate medical breakthrough that should not be sullied by shady operators. There are those in the 'fat industry,' who make their living from touting various 'fad diets,' who would love to ban HCG usage. Don't help their case.

They are more interested in treating the symptoms and selling supplements and multiple medications to the chronically obese... than curing them forever. Beware.

I am not a medical doctor, but I do have enough common sense to know that you are messing with a **critical part of your brain** that controls all of your body processes.

Do you want to **be victorious** and get control of your obesity? Find yourself an **enlightened doctor** directed program. Your **HCG supplies** should come from a **legitimate local pharmacy**.

Untangling the 'Worldwide Web'

The computer revolution is over... they won!

A lot of stuff on the internet is 'junk' and even obscene. However the positive side of the **computer revolution** and the world wide web is the tremendous access to information. Lots and lots of it. Many of you likely discovered **this tool kit** in that way.

The purpose of this section is to help you use the 'web' as an efficient tool to support and complement your HCG Victory Tool Kit. To that end I have weeded out and found some helpful websites for you. This not an exhaustive list, but it is the essence of what can be helpful for you and I. Remember, **we are after simpler**... not harder.

Basically there are three areas to look at: **(1)** general food Information, **(2)** products and brands, that I have tested and can recommend, **(3)** some 'local produce' locators.

What's the 'skinny' on What We eat.

You can find out just about anything about food these days. You don't need to learn how to build a 'clock' ...just how to use one properly to your advantage.

Here's **a few sites** I find helpful and **a brief summary** of the content.

You **do not need** all of **this information** to be victorious with your **doctor** directed **HCG diet plan**. But for those of you who want the, "...rrrrest of the story," as Paul Harvey used to say, here you go.

ISBN 978-0-9800641-7-9

Section Six: 'www' Food Information

Look before You Leap.

A **word** to the **wise**.

Don't be sucked into any kind of 'paid program' or allow yourself to be distracted from your **HCG program**. Keep your **focus** and you will be just fine.

More than one fitness or nutrition 'expert' have 'dissed' the HCG idea, only to 'eat their words' later. In my opinion 99% of them either **have never heard of it**, or have just been taught a certain method for 'their practice,' and have their 'blinders' in place.

Yes, this includes **some doctors** and **government bureaucrats**. When it comes to your **advisors**, **trainers** or **physicians**, find someone with **an open mind** that is **enlightened** and can **think independently**. Get yourself an **ally not a critic**.

"Keep your focus and you will be just fine."

General Food Information:

www.fns.usda.gov/fsn/

Your tax dollars at work. A kind of an umbrella site that allows you to research to your hearts content. Lots of background information and not a lot of 'spin.'

www.oph-good-housekeeping.com/food-nutrition.html

I like the searchable content by food categories, which allows you to look up an item (i.e. 'Fruits' and get a rundown by Calories, fat, carbs, protein and Nutritional value. Also has a good Q and A. section. I rate them fairly neutral.

Organic Foods:

www.eatwild.com

Information and sources for 'grass fed' beef, poultry, pork and dairy foods. Also for the adventurous... bison! (that would be buffalo to most of us) By the way buffalo is very good for you if you can find it locally. A commercial site.

"...find someone with an open mind that is enlightened and can think independently."

www.organic-center.org

Pro organic stance and funded by natural food producers. Very knowledge-able site with lots of insight into the value of organic foods and methods.

www.organicvalley.coop/

Another commercial site sponsored by organic food producers. Has a very good searchable, storehouse of data and research, on both the reasons to 'eat organic' and 'avoid non-organic' foods. Impressive content.

Section Six: 'www' Food Information

Recommended Products & Food Sources

Here is a short list of product brands I have **tested and used** and found to be great quality, tasty and very usable in the various phases of the diet.

"...brands I have tested and used and found to be great quality, tasty and usable in the various phases of the diet."

Table K Tested Foods Companies by Website Address			
www.site	Products for: HCG + 500	NS/NS	Life
www.Annie'sNaturals.com	YES	YES	YES
www.Bragg.com	YES	YES	YES
www.FrontierCoop.com	YES	YES	YES
www.GoodEarth.com	YES	YES	YES
www.OrganicVilleFoods.com	YES	YES	YES
www.TreeTop.com	YES	YES	YES
www.WildOrganics.net	YES	YES	YES

The list here is just a short one to get you started in the right direction.

Most all of them, not only are organic, but have links to other companies and co-op's that are in the same category. You will find a wide range of foods, seasonings and natural sweetening products that are HCG safe. It's a link to a whole new, safer world.

Some are financially supportive of organic farming and organic co-ops in the USA. So they put their money where their mouth is!

Local Produce Locators

The organic food issue begs the question... "Where can I get local organic food?"

www.LocavoreNetwork.com

"...find a local source for the type of produce you want, you can contact the farm through this site."

Odd name but a memorable one. This is the only comprehensive nation wide data base for over 15,000 farmers and the public sector. You can not only **find a local source** for the type of produce you want, you can **contact** the farm through this site. New and creating a lot of excitement. Holy cow!

Even includes **proper etiquette** to use when visiting a farm. Started out as one 'produce loving' man's hobby and mushroomed. **Interesting**.

ISBN 978-0-9800641-7-9

Section Seven:

'Taking the Next Step.'

"...it occurred to me that the change in shape could only be explained by a movement of fat away from abnormal deposits..."

Dr. A.T.W. Simeons

Defeat OBESITY...Forever!

The HCG Assisted 500 Calorie Weight Loss Cure

Section Seven: **PLANNING Your Next Step**

So Who is in Charge?

After you have reached your pounds and inches goals you are ready to move into the next phase of your HCG plan. You must **reset your body's natural weight management system**. You have to **take control** of this system and **re-train** it.

"You have to take control of this system and retrain it."

Remember the hypothalamus? Well it's still there and it remembers your pre HCG body weight. And so... guess what? It will immediately begin to move your body back to it's formerly obese self. But wait! Don't panic, the good doctor knows what to do.

Setting Your New Body Weight.

The proper method for ending your **HCG + 500 Calorie** phase of the diet is to continue on your 500 Calorie eating plan for **3 full days** after your **last HCG dose**.

Weigh yourself on the morning of the last day. Write it down on your "**No Sugar No Starch 7 Day Meal Planner.'** You will find it in **the pages that follow.**

Now you will begin an exercise to teach your body the correct weight you want to maintain from here on out. Just about everyone, no matter how much they know about dieting, nutrition, etc., thinks they will start to gain the weight back!

Relax. You can **keep it off successfully** if you follow the plan and stay on course. I was skeptical... but, it worked for me just like the doctor said. It will work for you, too!

How Sweet it... Isn't.

It is a good news, bad news scenario. The good news? For 21 days you can eat just about anything. What's the bad news? You must deny yourself **ALL SUGARS** and **STARCHES** during that time. It's just 3 weeks. You can do it.

"You must deny yourself ALL SUGARS and STARCHES during that time."

Here's the plan:

1) Your weight on the morning of your last HCG day, that you wrote down on your NO Sugar NO Starch meal planner... that is your **weight set point**. In my case it was 192.2 pounds.

2) You must return to a normal for you, daily caloric input, **without** the **sugars and starches**. (see 'Weights & Measures' page 61-65)

3) If your **daily morning weight** goes over your **weight set point** by even **one tenth** of a pound, you must IMMEDIATELY do a course correction. My action point was, 192.2 + 2.1 = 194.3 (2.1 over). See how that works?

Keep Your Bearings & Stay on Course.

Follow the **NO SUGAR/NO STARCH** rule and you will succeed in maintaining your weight. Be very careful, the **slightest** amount of either one, can knock you off course.

'Houston... We Have a Problem'

Once again this is important, if you find yourself **even one tenth of a pound** over the **2 pound** limit. Take corrective action **that very day**. You must **get back on course**.

Section Seven: **PLANNING Your Next Step**

Hooray! Hooray! For 'Steak Day!'

Here's **the answer**. You **fast all day**. No breakfast, no lunch, then for dinner eat a **huge, lean beef steak**. What do I mean by 'huge?' 12 to 16 ounces.

With your steak, you may have an apple and some tomatoes (or organic, no sugar ketchup) Remember to drink your liquids without limit. Cold or hot drinks curb hunger.

You will probably find yourself, up emptying your bladder more than usual that night. You will be rewarded in the morning. **'Poof'** the **extra pounds will be gone**.

I found that I needed one steak day a week to keep within the 2 lb. limit, during the 21 day stretch. So don't panic if you need a 'steak day' to get back on track. It's normal.

You are now in charge of your body's weight management system, and you never have to go back to the obesity lifestyle' again. You are probably healthier as a result.

"You must take corrective action that very day."

The 'Bell Lap.'

In every distance race there is a tradition of bell ringing that tells the runners that the end is in sight. The final stretch is just around the corner... **victory is coming**.

Hopefully you have run a good race. And victory is in your hands. After 21 days your new weight point is set. You are in charge of your weight at last and can start returning to a fairly normal, and hopefully improved, daily diet. Remember your calories.

Return to Earth

"...you never have to go back to the obesity lifestyle' again."

The final stage is to return to a **normal diet**, or as I like to call it 'return to earth and leave the fat behind' It's back to a normal diet, slowly adding the starches and sugars back in there... **slowly**. Be aware and in control of the Calories you are eating.

You really can eat a lot and stay at your weight set point. Be sure that you do, and you will eat healthier and more nutritious foods that give your body the balance it needs.

Your Fat Warehouse... Gone but not Forgotten.

You will find it **easier to eat less** and to **eat smarter**. Each of us has our achilles heel. You know your's. Remember your **fat warehouse** was established by your body to have a place to put the **'excess'** calories, so be aware of your **daily Calories**.

"You really can eat a lot and stay at your weight set point."

'Taking the Next Step'

You will find, starting on page 179, the **'See-Food Diet'** with **simplified food tables** and a **simplified list of Caloric choices** in the **No Sugar/No Starch** phase.

Also available for use with this tool kit is the **'HCG Victory Planner,'** a compilation of **already prepared master menus** with daily targets from **1200 to 2500** Calories. As well as **a plentiful supply** of the forms found in the **'HCG Victory Tool Kit.'**

Super Simeons 'Recipes for Victory.'

This is the third volume in the set and contains a compilation of **delicious** and **nutritious recipes and ideas** for all **three phases** of the **HCG protocol** including maintaining your **new life style** and your **new body**... for the rest of your life.

See the back of this book or our website: www.HCGVictoryToolKit.com

NO SUGAR NO STARCH ZONE

NO SUGAR & NO STARCH ZONE

FOOD... for Thought?

"Not all Calories are out in the open..."

Food... for Thought?

On any **average day** we are assaulted without mercy by...Calories! Yikes!

Have you noticed when you are in a grocery store the **most tempting** and **sugar laden**, **fat-laced** foods are right **at eye level**. That is **not an accident**.

Not all **Calories** are out in the open. Visualize this. You walk into the coffee shop and are faced with two temptations. Should you have that **jelly donut** or... the 'healthy' **raisin bran muffin**? Mmmm! Well of course you make the **healthy choice** and opt for the muffin... and **double** the Calories! **Ambushed again!**

It has been estimated by people, who sit around and keep track of such stuff, that we are exposed to **3000 to 4000 Calories** per day. Check the Calorie targets on page 64-65, and you will **notice something**. That would be about an **extra 1500 to 2000 Calories more** than most of us need... except for maybe someone named Michael. You know Michael Jordan or Michael Phelps.

That's **how we got into trouble** packing away all of that **fat in our warehouse.** An **extra 1500 Calories per day** adds about **12 lbs a year** to our 'storage facility.'

"...insanity is repeating the same thing over and over and expecting different results..."

Spoiled by 'Success'

Remember old Albert, who said, "...insanity is **repeating** the **same thing** over and over and **expecting different results**..." Our health and obesity problems grew out of our 'success' in finding and consuming **too many Calories**... which adds to our girth and **requires more**... you guessed it... CALORIES.

Defeating & controlling Your Obesity

If you have **followed this protocol honestly** and with all of **your determination** under a **physicians care**. If your **HCG was pure** and from a **legitimate pharmacy**. You should be **a lot lighter now!**

I lost **55 pounds** in **63 days** and I am **keeping it off**. Most likely, **you can too.**

You **never** have to go back. **You are almost free.**

"...you should be a lot lighter now!"

More Tools for Victory.

In the pages that follow you will find: **'Tips & Tricks,'** the **'See-Food Diet Plan,'** with easy to use approved **'Food Tables,'** and Charts for setting your Calorie **'targets,'** and also a complete set of **'No Sugar No Starch 7 Day Menu Planners.'**

Making Your 7 Day Meal Menu Plan

Follow the **instructions** and use the **tables** and **tips** that follow in this **'Tool-Kit'** and you will have every chance to **be victorious**.

Section Seven: **Some Tips & Tricks**

Measuring & Estimating Portions

If you want to carry around a set of measuring cups, you certainly could, but for most of us, it's just not practical. Here is **a list of sizes** and some **familiar objects** to help you **easily learn portion estimating** on the fly. You may find this very helpful.

"...easily learn portion estimating on the fly."

Just HOW BIG is...	...COMPARED TO these familiar items.
1 Teaspoon (tsp)	Same size as the TIP of your INDEX FINGER.
1 Tablespoon (TBSP)	Same size as the TOP half of your THUMB.
1/2 Cup	Half the Size of your balled FIST is a good guide.
1 Cup	The Size of your balled FIST is a good guide.
1 Medium Fruit	Same size as a BASEBALL.
1 oz. Cheese	Same size as your THUMB is a good guide.
3 oz. of MEAT	Same size as a deck of cards
6 oz. of MEAT	Same size as TWO decks of cards

A Simple Method for Your Plan

Try these suggestions, to easily arrive at your No Sugar/No Starch **weight setting menu**, more quickly and confidently. Pull out your **HCG + 500 Calorie** menu.

Okay we know that this is **a tested and proven plan**, using a 500 Calorie daily limit. All of the **foods** and the **rotation** in which you ate them has passed the test.
Your body and your palate are accustomed to it. You know it well.

"Why throw away all of that research?"

Why Re-invent the Wheel?

Why throw away all of that research? Use your **HCG + 500 Calorie menu** as the framework for **your NEW Menu**. Best to work in pencil. Try these suggestions:

Enlarging Your Calorie Count... the Easy way.	
First.	DOUBLE the PORTIONS which doubles the SAFE Calories
Second.	Carefully ADD some NEW 'SEE-FOOD' CHOICES to hit your target
Third.	Once you have a PLAN for 7 days just repeat it 3 times.

The 'SEE-FOOD' Diet Plan.

This section is your simplified 'SEE-FOOD' Diet Plan for the **3 Week NO SUGAR/NO STARCH Phase**. Aren't you sick of those big charts and complicated tables? Things don't have to be that complicated or comprehensive. Not when you have this 'tool kit' in your hands.

Here's how it works... if you **DON'T SEE IT** listed in this section... **DON'T EAT IT**!

It's Only 3 Weeks!

If you want to **succeed** in setting your bodies **new weight set point**, now that you have lost all that weight, it is VERY IMPORTANT that you **avoid sugars/starches** of any kind and keep your **weight within 2 pounds** of your final HCG day weight. **Review page 44** for the over-all plan.

'Simple Simeons' Works.

The **charts** that follow are admittedly 'mainstream' food items. You won't find page after page of fine print about the foods you cannot eat... instead you will find, only the **common garden variety** choices, totally safe and legal for this part of your HCG plan. So try to fight that urge for an 'ostrich steak' or 'exotic' fruit or veggie. You can deny yourself for three weeks. **Let's keep it simple and straightforward**.

Be sure to use the charts found on the following pages to plan & **record your strategy** and then just carefully follow your plan for three weeks. Look at the sample of my plan and you will get the idea. As I shared earlier, I just came up with **a one week plan,** and repeated it 3 times. Keep it simple and win.

The 'C' Word.

Yea, I know we are all a little sick of having **'Calories'** preached at us. Especially by some wiry little fitness 'guru' (choose your favorite). I suspect, most of them, have never been obese.

You **already know more**, about the **three types of fat** we carry around, and how to eliminate the 'abnormal' (warehoused fat), than most of them. When it comes to **Dr. Simeons weight loss cure** they are clueless. Don't let their pretense of superiority stop you... trust me, they will eat their words.

Show me just one of them who has lost 50 to 100 lbs. Show me the pictures... before and after.

'Fill'er Up... with High-Octane.

The most **common challenge** in **the No Sugar/NO Starch phase** is to **eat enough** Calories!

As the **HCG effect leaves** your body you **will not** be able to continue on 500 Calories a day... don't kid yourself, and don't let your over enthusiasm throw you off course. **Starvation does not work!**

You need to have a **general idea** of the correct range of **daily Calories required** for your final body weight. Remember **your body's system** will **try to go back** to where you were before the HCG cure.

Follow the Old Doctor's Plan... it Works!

First you need to determine the **correct Calorie consumption** for your weight, sex and frame size.

Your **doctor** can help here as well, but, based on some of the most up to date information, here's a guide to follow. Remember **you must eat enough** and keep the **protein up** and the **balance** that you had on the 500 Calorie menu.

A quick review: 40% protein, 30% fruits, 30% vegetables seems to be **a very successful ratio**.

Notice... **NO sugar or sugar additives or NO starch or starch laden products**.

The best sharpshooters in the world can't hit the bullseye if they can't see the target. Use the information on the charts that follow to describe your **'Daily Calorie bullseye.'** This is step one.

Need to Review?

Revisit pages 61-65 and take another look at the weight ranges and **frame sizes**. we will use the same terminology in the 'Calorie Targets.' Your goal is to **maintain** your new weight, **not** lose weight.

At the top of page 64 is **a simple method** for determining your frame size.

Be sure to **use your NEW Weight** on the tables. Remember, your new weight, is how much you weighed on your final HCG day. You are going to keep your **daily weight strictly within TWO pounds** of that number. If you start to wander you will immediately utilize **a 'steak day'** to correct course.

OK, now you should be **ready to check the chart** below and find your 'Calorie bullseye' and write it down on your **'NO Sugar & Starch 7 Day Meal Planner'** found on pages 187-191. **Ladies first.**

Daily Calorie Targets for LADIES: Average Activity

Frame Size	TOTAL Calories	(40% Protein)	(30% Fruit)	(30% Veg)	NOTES:
Small Frame	1400	(560)	(420)	(420)	Average Activity
Medium Frame	1500	(600)	(450)	(450)	Average Activity
Large Frame	1600	(640)	(480)	(480)	Average Activity

A Simple Adjustment for Lifestyle.

To stay true to **the principles of simplicity** we are following in this **'HCG Victory Tool Kit'** I have studied the available material from internet advisory sources such as the (ADA) American Diabetes Association, among many others and boiled it down to a simple rule of thumb for setting these targets. My solution is to add a **'Lifestyle' adjustment table**. **Age adjustments** for men are also noted.

Close Does Count in 'Horseshoes' and 'Calories.'

It's good to keep in mind, that our bodies are all variations of the **same thing** but **different**, and so some **adjustments** are okay. That is why **keeping good records is so important**. Knowing how we react to different foods and how our weight is affected is critical, because some **course corrections are inevitable**. The first principle of navigation is that **you must know exactly** where you are **and** how you got there, only then can you **correct your course** or find your way back. **You can do it.**

Remember in this phase we are **shooting for a bullseye** with a 10% margin for accuracy. It is better to eat a little too much and then dial it back than to starve out and wobble off course.

Simple ADJUSTMENTS for Lifestyle: LADIES : LOW Activity

Small Frame	-100	(520)	(390)	(390)	LOW Activity
Medium Frame	-150	(540)	(405)	(405)	LOW Activity
Large Frame	-200	(560)	(420)	(420)	LOW Activity

Simple ADJUSTMENTS for Lifestyle: LADIES: VERY Active

Small Frame	+100	(600)	(450)	(450)	VERY Active
Medium Frame	+150	(660)	(495)	(495)	VERY Active
Large Frame	+200	(720)	(540)	(540)	VERY Active

Doing The Math.

An example: **Medium Frame** with **Low Activity** level: (1500 C - 150 C = **1350 Calories Daily Target**

Daily Calorie Targets for MEN: AVERAGE ACTIVITY

Frame Size	TOTAL Calories	(40% Protein)	(30% Fruit)	(30% Veg)	NOTES:
Small Frame	1800/1600	(720/640)	(540/480)	(540/480)	Average Activity
Medium Frame	2000/1800	(800/720)	(600/540)	(600/540)	Average Activity
Large Frame	2300/2000	(920/800)	(690/600)	(690/600)	Average Activity

Men and the Age Factor.

Sources such as the American Diabetes Association (ADA) usually factor in men's ages more than women as far as Caloric requirements. In plain english, that means we as a group for a variety of reasons, on average add more fat as we grow older, than women do. It just seems to be a fact of life.

So the 'adjustment tables for men' reflect that 'age factor' in the following ways.

You will see **two figures** in each column (i.e. 1800/1600) the first figure is for men **under age 60** the second is **for those of us over 60**. That seems to be the most common dividing line. Of course there are exceptions. Your personal physician knows. Remember, this is a **doctor directed protocol**.

'Horseshoes' and 'Calories.'

Once again, remember in this phase we are **shooting for a bullseye** with a 10% margin for accuracy. It is better to eat a little too much and then dial it back than to starve out and wobble off course.

Simple ADJUSTMENTS for Lifestyle and Age: LOW ACTIVITY

Small Frame	-100	(680/600)	(510/450)	(510/450)	LOW Activity
Medium Frame	-200	(720/640)	(540/480)	(540/480)	LOW Activity
Large Frame	-300	(800/680)	(600/510)	(600/510)	LOW Activity

Simple ADJUSTMENTS for Lifestyle and Age: VERY ACTIVE

Small Frame	+150	(780/700)	(585/525)	(585/525)	VERY Active
Medium Frame	+200	(880/700)	(660/600)	(660/600)	VERY Active
Large Frame	+250	(1020/900)	(765/675)	(765/675)	VERY Active

Doing Your Math Homework.

Okay guys, here's a few simple examples... it's not rocket science: **Use the first set of numbers if you are under age 60, the second numbers if you are 'seasoned.'**

> **UNDER age 60.**
>
> **Medium Frame** with **Low Activity** level: (C = 2000 - 200 C = **1800 Calories Daily.**
>
> **Medium Frame** with **VERY Active** level: (C = 2000 + 200 C = **2200 Calories Daily.**
>
> **OVER age 60.**
>
> **Medium Frame** with **Low Activity** level: (C = 1800 - 200 C = **1600 Calories Daily.**
>
> **Medium Frame** with **VERY Active** level: (C = 1800 + 200 C = **2000 Calories Daily.**

Section Seven: The 'SEE-FOOD' Planner

Don't SEE IT... Don't Eat it...that's the PLAN!

You should have your total Calorie targets set and you should now be ready to start building your seven day plan. This is step two. Look in the pages that follow, find your form entitled **'No Sugar or Starch 7 day Menu Planner.'** It's okay to remove the page from the book or copy it for your own personal use. (See page 197 for more resources)

Write your **daily targets** at the top in the space provided. Note that the **Calorie balance** of **protein**, **fruits** and **vegetables is noted** at the bottom of each column. Use that number as a goal.

The **'Menu Selections'** are in alphabetical order by category and within each category. Carbs are noted, sugar is not, because any 'natural' sugar that is an integral part of the food selections originally approved by Dr. Simeons, can normally be consumed in this step, without a problem.

DRINKS: 3 Week-No Sugar/Starch Phase

Water, Water Everywhere...

Okay this is a good place to start. Getting **plenty of liquids** is, as always, important for your health. Not a lot of Calories to worry about if you follow the chart. No sugars or dairy products added. 68 ounces.

Description	Serving Size	Calories	Protein	Fiber	Carbs	Notes:
COFFEE	8 oz	0	0	0	0	Black
LEMON JUICE, Fresh	4 oz	30	0	0	10	
LIME JUICE, Fresh	8 oz	30	1	0	10	
TOMATO JUICE	4 oz	20	1	0	5	
V-8 JUICE	4 oz	25	1	1	5	
WATER, Pure	8 oz	0	0	0	0	No Limit

DAIRY PRODUCTS: 3 Week-No Sugar/Starch Phase

Making the Most with the Least.

You can use these two **Dairy based products** to augment your recipes and add variety and some safe Calories to your daily plan. Remember to keep the **variety and rotation** going.

Note that the pudding choice here may contain **aspartame** as a sweetner. You will have to decide. We are only talking about **a three week period** and the pudding does fill in the 'dessert' slot. Helps fill the 'chocolate' void and is fat free and low calorie. There are **some reasonable trade-offs** there.

Description	Serving Size	Calories	Protein	Fat	Sat Fat	Notes:
COTTAGE CHEESE, Small Curd	4 TBSP	60	0	0	0	Black
PUDDING, Fat Free-Sugar Free	4 oz	70	0	0	0	Milk

FRUITS: 3 Week-No Sugar/Starch Phase

Expanding Your Fruit Palette.

Now you can start adding more fruits to your meals. Add new flavors and great eye appeal. Safe way to bulk up your Calories. Keep good records and watch the balance and rotation.

Description	Serving Size	Calories	Protein	Fiber	Carbs	Notes:
APPLES	1 med.	70	0	3	19	Organic*
APPLESAUCE-Unsweetened	3 oz	35	0	1	11	
BLACKBERRIES	1 Cup	55	0	2	14	Raw
BLUEBERRIES	1 Cup	40	1	4	11	Raw
CRANBERRIES, Dried	2 Tbsp	44	0	1	12	No sugar
GRAPEFRUIT	1/2 med	60	1	4	14	
RASPBERRIES	1 Cup	50	1	3	13	Raw
STRAWBERRIES	1 Cup	68	1	5	16	Raw
NECTARINES	1 med	70	1	1	16	Organic*
PEACHES	1 med	38	1	1	9	Organic*
PLUMS	1 med	30	0	2	8	Organic*
TANGERINES	1 med	50	1	2	14	Organic*

MEAT & EGGS: 3 Week-No Sugar/Starch Phase

Add Lean Pork to Your Menu.

Continue to trim fat and weigh raw, keeping in mind your protein balance and increased Caloric needs.

Description	Serving Size	Calories	Protein	Fiber	Carbs	Notes:
EGGS, Poached	1 Large	76	6	0	0	No OIL
BACON	1 slice	34	2	0	0	
BEEF, Lean Steak	4 oz	150	25	0	0	Page 57
BEEF, Roast	1 oz	170	24	0	0	
CHICKEN, Breast-Broiled/Baked	4 oz	70	14	2	2	Skinless
FISH, Low Fat-Baked/Broiled	4 oz	90	30	0	0	Page 58
PORK CHOPS, Lean Center Cut	3 oz	150	20	0	0	Trimmed
TURKEY/CHICKEN, Hot Dog	1 dog	100	6	0	1	
SHRIMP, broiled/barbequed	3 oz	100	20	0	0	No Sauce

VEGETABLE TALES: 3 Week-No Sugar/Starch Phase

A Great Supporting Cast

Not a lot of Calories here. So you may find it challenging to keep your veggies up in the 30% range of your daily plan. The good news is you can eat these like crazy. Keep good records, because as previously mentioned, tomatoes can be a problem for some people. I was one of those. This gives you a lot more vegetables for your rotation. Also you can start mixing them in your salads and meals.

Description	Serving Size	Calories	Protein	Fiber	Carbs	Notes:
ALFALFA SPROUTS	1/2 Cup	5	1	1	1	Salad
ASPARAGUS	4 oz	25	3	2	0	Steamed
BROCCOLI	1 Cup	44	5	5	6	Steamed
BRUSSEL SPROUTS	1 Cup	38	3	3	8	Steamed
CABBAGE	4 oz	28	1	1	6	Salad
CARROTS, Cooked or Raw	1/2 Cup	30	1	2	6	
CELERY	1 Cup	18	1	2	4	Raw
CHERRY TOMATOES	1 Cup	28	1	2	3	Salad
CUCUMBERS, 'Larry size'	1 Cup	16	1	1	3	Salad
EGGPLANT	1 Cup	35	1	2	9	
GREEN BEANS, Cooked	1 Cup	38	2	4	8	
LETTUCE, All Varieties	1 Cup	20	2	2	0	Salad
MUSHROOMS	4 med	15	2	0	3	Salad
ONIONS, Green RAW	1 Cup	25	1	1	1	Chopped
ONIONS, Red, Yellow, White	1 Cup	30	1	1	7	Trimmed
PEPPERS, Hot Chili-red/green	1 med	15	1	1	3	Salad
PEPPERS, Bell-All Colors	1 Cup	30	1	1	7	Salad
RADISHES, Raw	1 Cup	30	1	1	1	Salad
SPINACH, Raw	1 Cup	12	1	0	0	Salad
SPINACH, COOKED	1 Cup	42	5	0	0	

Setting Up Your Plan.

Okay, time to go to work and put your **SEVEN day NO SUGAR/NO STARCH** menu plans together.

On the following pages you will find the **forms you need** to do that. Only this time, to set your body's weight at the goal you have achieved, you are developing a **three week long plan.** Note that the 'menu plan' has room for seven days. **Remember** you can use your 5 day plan as a foundation for this one, **making the necessary adjustments**. A good approach is to do a great one week plan and repeat it 3 times. This is the next step.

Section Seven: **The 7 Day NO Sugar NO Starch MENU**

Setting Your Body's NEW Weight.

The critical part of **keeping your new weight** is to keep it within **two pounds** of your weight on your last HCG day. Now it's **time to plan** your meals around your new Caloric needs (pages 180-181) and set your course and stay on it. Below and on the next page is a partial copy of the '**HCG + 500 Calorie 7 Day Meal Planner**.

"...it's time to plan your meals around the 500 Calorie plan"

"I found the best approach was to pre-plan the meals using the Food Tables found at the beginning of this chapter."

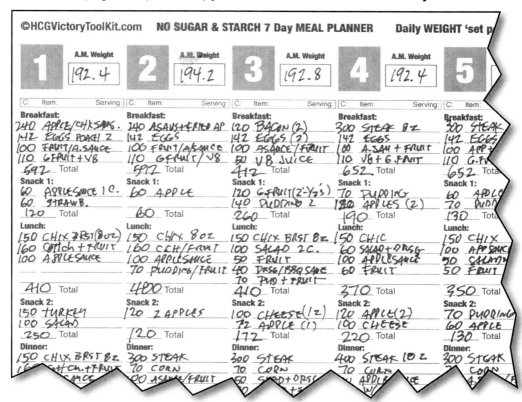

Simplicity is the Keyword in this 'Tool Kit.'

I found the best approach was to **pre-plan** the meals using the **Food Tables** found in the '**See-Food Tables.**' With the use of these tables, carefully put together your daily meals. It may help to **review** the pages on '**The 500 Calorie + HCG Diet**' found at the beginning of '**Section Three: Your Plan for Victory.**' (pages 40-44)

In the pages ahead, you will find **3 copies**, of the one sided form above. Each one covers **7 days**, which matches the three week length, of this **NO Sugar/NO Starch phase**. Before you use all of the forms go ahead and **make some blank copies**, for **your personal use**. See how I completed the form above.

"Once you have a few 5 day plans that you have tested and you like you can just repeat them as often as needed..."

A time saver is to just use your **HCG 5 day plan** as a **frame work** and make the necessary adjustments, then **repeat** your selections being careful to **alternate and rotate** your protein, fruit, and vegetable choices.

Once you have a **7 day plan perfected** that you have tested and like, you can just **repeat** it two more times. Be sure that the 'Day 7' and 'Day 1' choices are **not** the same. For example, be sure the last protein for Day 7 and the first one for 'Day 1' aren't the same. **Keep the rotation going.**

Section Seven: **The 7 Day NO Sugar NO Starch MENU**

Watching Your Daily Weight.

Below is a partial copy of the '**NO Sugar/NO Starch 7 Day Meal Planner**' showing the left side and bottom. You will note that I didn't hit the **2000 Calorie** goal exactly each day, which is okay, but I did keep my '**Daily WEIGHT Set Point**' on target.

"...it's time to plan your meals around the 500 Calorie plan

"I found the best approach was to pre-plan the meals using the Food Tables found at the beginning of this chapter."

"Once you have a few 5 day plans that you have tested and you like you can just repeat them as often as needed..."

MEAL PLANNER   **Daily WEIGHT 'set point' Target:** _192.2_   **Daily CALORIE TARGET:** _2000_

	Day 4 (192.4)	Day 5 (191.0)	Day 6 (191.2)	Day 7 (191.2)
A.M. Weight	192.8			
Breakfast:	300 STEAK 8z / 142 EGGS / 100 A.SAU + FRUIT / 110 V8 + G.FRUIT — Total 652	300 STEAK / 142 EGGS 2 / 100 APP + FRUIT / 110 G.FRUIT + V8 — Total 652	FRIED 240 A.SAUSAGE APPLES / 142 2 EGGS / 100 A.SAUCE/FRUIT / 110 G.FRUIT + V8 — Total 592	140 A.SAUS + APPLES / 142 EGGS / 100 A.SAUCE + FRUIT / 110 G.FRUIT + V8 — Total 592
Snack 1:	70 PUDDING / 180 APPLES (2) — Total 190	60 APPLE / 70 PUDDING — Total 130	60 APPLE / 70 PUDDING — Total 130	60 APPLE / 70 PUDDING — Total 130
Lunch:	150 CHIC / 60 SALAD + DRSG / 100 APPLESAUCE / 60 FRUIT — Total 370	150 CHIX / 100 APP SAUCE / 50 SALAD + DRSG / 50 FRUIT — Total 350	150 CHIX SALAD / 100 APPLES / 180 COTT CH/S.BERRY / 50 3/4 cup — Total 480	150 CHIX / 110 APPLE + G.RN SAL / 80 COTT CH + STRAWB — Total 440
Snack 2:	120 APPLE (2) / 100 CHEESE — Total 220	70 PUDDING / 60 APPLE — Total 130	70 PUDDING / 160 APP + CHEESE — Total 230	160 CHEES + APPLE / 70 PUDDING — Total 230
Dinner:	400 STEAK 10z / 70 CORN / 100 APPLESAUCE w/ FRUIT / 70 PUDDING (1) — Total 640	300 STEAK / 70 CORN / A.SAUCE/FRUIT / 100 COFFEE/LATTE (NO SUGAR) — Total 470	300 STEAK / 70 CORN / 150 SALAD w TOM/APP — Total 520	300 STEAK / 50 SM SALAD / 180 COTT CHEESE/FRUIT — Total 530
Snack 3:	200 APPLE w/ CHEESE / 70 PUDDING (1) — Total 270	200 APP + CHEESE / 70 PUDDING — Total 270	120 APP + ORANGE / 70 PUDDING — Total 190	200 APPL + CHEESE / 100 PUDDING/FRUIT — Total 300
Notes: Protein:	850 + CHEES.	+ EGGS 750 CHSE	630 + EGGS + CHEESE	EGGS 630 CHEESE
Fruits:				
Veggies:				
TODAY'S TOTAL	2342	2002	2142	2222.

Watch the 2 POUND Limit & Everything Will Be Fine.

You don't have to hit your Calories exactly, remember it is a target to shoot for. The only number you must be precise on, is your morning weight. Be sure to be consistent with time of day, what you're wearing, the scale (when traveling take it). Immediate action is required. Do the '**steak day**' that very day. (page 174 & 196)

You should be **experiencing the joy** and **amazement** that we all go through.

NO SUGAR & STARCH 7 Day MEAL PLANNER

Daily WEIGHT 'set point' Target:

Daily CALORIE TARGET:

	1	2	3	4	5	6	7
A.M. Weight							

Each day column contains:

C: | Serving: | Item:

Breakfast:

_____ Total

Snack 1:

_____ Total

Lunch:

_____ Total

Snack 2:

_____ Total

Dinner:

_____ Total

Snack 3:

_____ Total

Notes:
Protein:
Fruits:
Veggies:

TODAY'S TOTAL

NO SUGAR & STARCH 7 Day MEAL PLANNER

Daily WEIGHT 'set point' Target: _____

Daily CALORIE TARGET: _____

	Day 1	Day 2	Day 3	Day 4	Day 5	Day 6	Day 7
A.M. Weight	☐	☐	☐	☐	☐	☐	☐

Column labels per day: **C:** | **Item:** | **Serving:**

Meal		
Breakfast:		
		Total ____
Snack 1:		
		Total ____
Lunch:		
		Total ____
Snack 2:		
		Total ____
Dinner:		
		Total ____
Snack 3:		
		Total ____
Notes:		
Protein:		
Fruits:		
Veggies:		
		TODAY'S TOTAL ☐

©HCGVictoryToolKit.com   NO SUGAR & STARCH 7 Day MEAL PLANNER

Daily WEIGHT 'set point' Target: **Daily CALORIE TARGET:**

	Day 1	Day 2	Day 3	Day 4	Day 5	Day 6	Day 7
A.M. Weight							
Serving: / C: / Item:							
Breakfast:							
Total							
Snack 1:							
Total							
Lunch:							
Total							
Snack 2:							
Total							
Dinner:							
Total							
Snack 3:							
Total							
Notes:							
Protein:							
Fruits:							
Veggies:							
TODAY'S TOTAL							

TROUBLE SHOOTING:

NOTES & RESOURCES

TROUBLE SHOOTING:

Section Seven: **Trouble Shooting TIPS & TECHNIQUES**

Problem:

" I seem to be 'stuck'... not gaining or losing...

What do I do?

Solutions:

"An 'apple-day' begins at lunch and continues until just before lunch of the following day..."

"...The 'apple-day' produces a gratifying loss of weight on the following day, chiefly due to the elimination of water..."

"Be sure to get adequate rest and enough sleep to avoid affecting your weigh loss..."

Dealing with 'Weight Plateaus'

If you have **followed the plan carefully**, hitting little pauses in your weight loss is **nothing** to be concerned about, There are **several possible causes**.

This is where your careful **record keeping**, yes, the ones I have been harping about, become an invaluable tool. Also a plateau is more likely during the **HCG + 500 Calorie** phase. Dr. Simeons reassures us, that it is simply a normal sequence of events. He also indicates that if you **stay the course** eventually you will break the plateau and continue to lose weight normally. (see page 137-138)

A plateau seems to be inevitable if you start out losing weight very quickly... and most of us do. Assuming you have not committed any dietary errors, if you are **stalled for 4-6 days**, here is what you should do;

    1) Check your menu plan for any errors.
    2) Check your seasoning, etc. for any hidden sugars or starches.
    3) Have you eaten any tomatoes, oranges or seafood?

You can consult with your doctor, but if **everything checks out** okay, you are probably having, what I like to call, a **'normal adjustment plateau.'** Here's why.

As you burn Calories from your stored fat, the **supporting tissues**, blood vessels, etc., that exist solely to service, that warehouse fat, remain. In a few days they will **be fully absorbed** into your body and your downward weight march will resume.

The **bonus** here, is that all of the vitamins and minerals, etc. in those tissues, is absorbed into **back into your system**, along with the **fat** and the **nutrients** in it.

The **exception** of course, is if you are about at the end of your HCG plan, and your supply of **warehouse fat** is **exhausted**. Consult with **your doctor**, to see for sure.

Dr. Simeons Pacifier... the 'Apple Day'

"An 'apple-day' begins at lunch and continues until just before lunch of the following day. The patients are given **six large apples** and are told to eat one whenever they feel the desire though six apples is the **maximum** allowed.

During an apple-day **no** other **food** or **liquids except plain water** are allowed and of water, they may only drink, if eating an apple still leaves them thirsty. Just enough to quench an uncomfortable thirst,

Most patients feel no need for water and are **quite happy** with their six apples.

The **apple-day** produces a gratifying loss of weight on the following day, chiefly due to the **elimination of water.** This water is not regained when the patients resume their normal 500-Calorie diet at lunch, and on the following days they continue to **lose weight** satisfactorily."

Check Your Exercise & Rest Cycles.

The good doctor does not see a huge benefit in rigorous exercise and recommends that **moderate** exercise is fine. Remember, you are targeting your 'stored fat.' Not the 'dynamic fat,' that your body taps into when stressed, and then replaces.

Not getting **adequate rest** and enough sleep will negatively affect your weight loss.

Section Seven: **Trouble Shooting TIPS & TECHNIQUES**

Problem:

"I am over the 2 pound limit on my weight setting phase...

...How Can I Fix That?"

Solutions:

"A 'steak day..."

"... fast all day. No breakfast, no lunch, then for dinner eat a huge lean beef steak..."

"Unless an adequate amount of protein is eaten as soon as the treatment is over, protein deficiency is bound to develop..."

No Sugar No Starch & The 2 pound Limit.

A critical part of your success in resetting your body's s weight management system to the new and improved weight you now have is the infamous '2 pound limit.'

If you exceed the 2 pound gain limit, you must immediately take corrective action.

The 'Steak Day' is the Answer.

Here's **the answer**. You fast all day. No breakfast, no lunch, then for dinner eat a huge lean beef steak. What do I mean by 'huge?' 12 to 16 ounces.

With your steak, you may have an apple and some tomatoes (or organic, no sugar ketchup) Remember to drink your liquids without limit. Cold or hot drinks curb hunger.

You will probably find yourself, up emptying your bladder more than usual that night. You will be rewarded in the morning. 'Poof' **the extra pounds** will be gone.

I found that I needed **one** steak day a week to keep within the 2 lb. limit, during the 21 day stretch. So don't panic if you need a 'steak day' to get back on track. It's normal.

You are now in charge of your body's weight management system, and you never have to go back to the obesity lifestyle' again. You are probably healthier as a result.

Protein Deficiency 'hunger - edema' Explained.

Once again, read what the good doctor has to say, about a common misconception.

"During treatment the patient has been only just above the verge of protein deficiency and has had the advantage of protein being fed back into his system from the breakdown of fatty tissue. Once the treatment is over there is no more HCG in the body and this process no longer takes place. Unless an **adequate** amount of **protein** is eaten as soon as the treatment is over, **protein deficiency** is bound to develop, and this inevitably causes the marked retention of water known as **hunger - edema**.

The treatment is very simple.

The patient is told to eat **two eggs** for **breakfast** and a **huge steak** for **lunch** and **dinner** followed by a large helping of **cheese** and to phone through the weight the next morning. When these instructions are followed a stunned voice is heard to report that **two lbs.** have **vanished overnight**, that the ankles are normal but that sleep was disturbed, owing to an extraordinary need **to pass large quantities of water.**

The patient having learned this lesson usually has no further trouble."

(Note: This is another version of the infamous 'steak day.')

www.HCGVictoryToolKit.com

Check our website for updates and additional resources.

Section Seven: | **HCG Victory BOOKS**

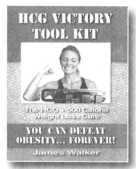

'HCG Victory
Tool Kit'
©2009

'HCG Victory Tool Kit'

A **comprehensive** and **easy to understand** guide for successfully winning your war with obesity. Clearly and carefully constructed to provide **maximum** help with a **minimum** of frustration. The book is really **four books in one** and indispensable.

It contains a complete road map and all of the food tables and recipes you need to succeed. Includes a generous supply of forms to plan, record and track your weight loss for the critical, '**HCG + 500 Calorie**' and '**No Sugar No Starch**' phases. A **bonus** is a completely new presentation of Doctor Simeons manuscript in an easier to read and understand **format**, with added table of contents and diagrams.

If you are serious about the HCG weight loss plan this is absolutely **the best book**.

$34.95 (8.25 x 11.0 inches, 200 pages) **ISBN 978-0-9800641-7-9**

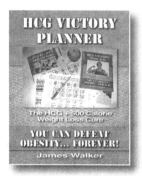

HCG Victory
Planner
©2009

'HCG Victory PLANNER'

By popular demand, a **companion volume** for use with the '**HCG Victory Tool Kit**'

All of the suggested menus for the '**HCG + 500 Calorie**' and the '**No Sugar No Starch**' phases are supplied. You will find **already filled out menu plans** for the 5 day and 7 day menu plans. Even contains a shopping list.

The 7 day plans come in 1200 to 2500 Calorie **pre-made plans** in 100 Calorie increments! **Just pick a menu and go.** A generous supply of all of the blank menu plans, charts and forms, are also included, so **no copying required!**

If you want a '**turn-key**' **solution** for your HCG weight loss plan and a proven track to run on, then this book is the addition you need to your '**Victory Collection.**'

$24.95 (8.25 x 11.0 inches, 100 pages) **ISBN 978-0-9800641-8-6**

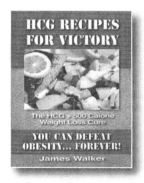

Super Simeons
'Recipes for
Victory'
©2010

'Super Simeons RECIPES for VICTORY'

A **full color companion volume** for use with the '**HCG Victory Tool Kit**'

A special collection of recipes for use with both the '**HCG + 500 Calorie**' and the '**No Sugar No Starch**' plans, as well as plenty of '**Return to Earth**' recipes for that trip back to **your new normal**. Full of mouth-watering **delicious** and **nutritious** recipes presented in **eye appealing full color!**

If you want **a library of recipes** for your HCG weight loss plan and your **new body** and **lifestyle**, then add this **super recipe book** to your '**Victory Collection.**'

$39.95 (8.25 x 11.0 inches, 200 pages) **ISBN 978-0-9800641-9-3**

Section Seven: **INSPIRATIONAL BOOKS by GreatNewsPress.Com**

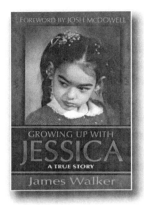

'Growing Up with JESSICA'
Second Edition
©July 2009

The 'Growing Up with JESSICA, Second Edition'

A **moving and inspirational true story**, told clearly and passionately by Jessica's father. Part mystery, part tragedy and 100% inspirational. The book is an honest sharing of the ups and downs of **an unexpected event** in the Walker family.

Shaken to the **very roots** of their faith, Jim & Renée and their family, found healing as they successfully grappled with every **parent's worst nightmare.**

Travel along with them as they experience the roller coaster ride of tragedy, love, hope and faith, growing up with Jessica. **You will emerge touched and inspired.**

$14.95 (5.5 x 8.5 inches, 204 pages) **ISBN 978-0-9800641-0-0**

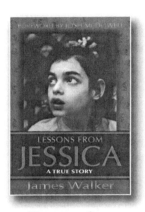

'Lessons from JESSICA'
©2010

'Lessons from JESSICA'

After publishing **'Growing up with Jessica.'** many readers began asking questions about the full spectrum and many **different facets** of our experience. At first we published a newsletter and then that newsletter evolved into this book.

It is designed to be a resource and guide, about the things we learned as we **'grew up with Jessica.'** At the end of each chapter are a few **'Questions for Further Thought'** and a **'Love-in-Action Point'** to help **apply the concepts.**

A **comforting,** encouraging, and enlightening book, for those facing life changing **affliction,** including their **friends and family,** who want to **be there** for them.

$14.95 (5.5 x 8.5 inches, 204 pages) **ISBN 978-0-9800641-1-7**

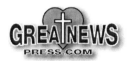

Our Mission:

Our mission and purpose is to offer books that do more than just motivate men, women and children... but **inspire** them. Inspiration takes many forms and has many applications.

" ...the action or power of moving the intellect or emotions..."
...the act of influencing or suggesting opinions..."

Inspirational Books by GreatNewsPress.com

Section Seven: List of Tables and Illustrations

Section Seven: **NOTES:**

Breinigsville, PA USA
25 April 2010
236766BV00001B/13/P